A STILL LIFE

A STILL LIFE

A Memoir

Josie George

BLOOMSBURY PUBLISHING

LONDON · OXFORD · NEW YORK · NEW DELHI · SYDNEY

BLOOMSBURY PUBLISHING
Bloomsbury Publishing Plc
50 Bedford Square, London, WC1B 3DP, UK
29 Earlsfort Terrace, Dublin 2, Ireland

BLOOMSBURY, BLOOMSBURY PUBLISHING and the Diana logo are
trademarks of Bloomsbury Publishing Plc

First published in Great Britain 2021

A catalogue record for this book is available from the British Library

ISBN: HB: 978-1-5266-1197-0; EBOOK: 978-1-5266-1201-4

2 4 6 8 10 9 7 5 3

Typeset by Newgen KnowledgeWorks Pvt., Ltd, Chennai, India
Printed and bound in Great Britain by CPI Group (UK) Ltd, Croydon CR0 4YY

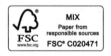

To find out more about our authors and books visit www.bloomsbury.com
and sign up for our newsletters

For all the women who led me right here

Prologue

I write this from my bed in an old terraced house that's seen out a hundred and fifty slow laps of the sun. I've spent the last fifteen of them here. Same old walls, same old view.

My compressed home is one room wide and riddled with damp. Sometimes I lie stretched out on the floor, taking up most of its width, and I think of it cheerfully relying on the houses either side of it to hold it up. It feels twice as strong than any reserved, detached affair because of it. When the wind blows, fierce and menacing, you can sit on the steep stairs between the two floors. You can close your eyes and feel the phrase 'safe as houses' as a holy, irrefutable truth.

Houses like mine exist all in a row along every street of my industrial West Midlands neighbourhood. They push themselves right up against the narrow pavement, rusty weeds marking the join. It's a land of scattered wheelie bins, patched grass, broken glass, dog shit and prowling cats. Cars ride the corners and the yellow lines because there is never anywhere to park. The neighbours shout behind closed doors and smile at you in the street, and for half the year the old people drag plastic garden chairs to sit outside their front doors and smoke in the sunshine, their heads tipped back to the sky. We're good to each other. We're so trodden together that we have to be. There is peace and reassurance in that and I like living here.

I share the house with my nine-year-old son and no one else. Our days follow a repetitive, quiet rhythm. I take him to school, him dutifully shifting each bin that blocks our path so I can squeeze past on my mobility scooter. We make up phrases beginning with the letters on the car number plates we see, each as daft as we can manage. 'Bee, ee, ess!' I call. 'Bubbly . . . elephant . . . *SNEEZES*!' he returns. We are happy with each other. I watch him run to his friends in the playground and then I go home again.

I write. I rest. Some days, when I'm well enough, I'll scoot to the community centre the next street over and write there for a while until I need to lie down again. I've spent the last few years trying to make a living with my words and thoughts. I don't really know what else to do.

I write the words, but often I won't say a sound out loud until it's time to pick up my son from school again. I don't mind it. There have always been long years when I've struggled to leave my house for more than an hour or two at a time and so I am used to solitude.

I am thirty-six years old.

The first thing you'll want to know, I expect, is what's wrong with me. That's always the first thing people ask, their eyes sliding to my legs, my slump, and so I will say now that I don't know. I don't know what's wrong with me. I've spent my whole life wondering too.

There seems to be something different about my body. It can't control its equilibrium: its weather. Movement, sensation and sensory input, circulation and cardiac control: my body responds wildly to any exertion, to adrenaline, to stimulation, to changes in temperature, to its own processes of digestion, blood flow and immunity. It is a bucking horse; a frightened, alien bird. My symptoms started in my babyhood, and so the 'what's wrong with you?' question is an old one. That's why I need to go back through my life to tell you this story. All the way back to the beginning.

These days, right now, I feel it as a squeezing, heavy pain from my waist down. My heart relies on pace-making drugs to stop it racing me into unconsciousness when I stand or move. All day long, my body lurches into responses of too little or too much in unpredictable, laughable ways. The hours fill up with extreme physical responses and with sudden, profound fatigue. Energy pours out from me: I can't keep it in. I will suddenly stop and crumple like a puppet with its strings cut and then I can't get up again. Activity, food, light, sound, stress, needing the toilet, even gravity, excitement, surprise, laughter, crying, fear. It sounds ridiculous and it is. All the normal aspects of a human life throw my nervous system into confusion and all have a cost; all hurt or overwhelm me. I can only ride it, ride my life, holding on, while I try to shape my days and my time into something more interesting and more dignified than all of this.

I move slowly through it. For the last few years, I've only been able to walk a dozen steps here and there. I don't understand why more is not possible, but more results in the kind of pain I can't talk through easily, lasting for hours, days; the kind that stops you dead. More results in exhaustion and tachycardia, sickness and unconsciousness and a cacophony of all my most unpleasant symptoms. I live around gentle bursts of choice and exertion, continually paced, evaluated, adjusted, every day a little different, every day new. Things haven't always been as bad as this, but they have been sometimes, before now. Like a wheel turning, there are times in my life when the grip of it loosens for a little while – at least, that's how it's worked before – it's just that before long, something takes hold again. I have learnt that this is simply how it is and that it's best to get on with life privately and quietly, to let progress and change happen slowly. You avoid too much judgement that way and there has often been plenty of that.

What I experience has been called many things over the years by different doctors at different times, depending on their speciality, what tests they run, and how they view bodies like mine: Dysautonomia, Postural Orthostatic Tachycardia Syndrome (POTS), M.E. or Chronic Fatigue Syndrome (CFS), Functional Neurological Disorder (FND), Functional Gastrointestinal Disorder (FGID), Sensory Processing Disorder.

I have learnt, with deep shame at times, that these names passed backwards and forwards down my medical history mean very little in any tangible sense and so I struggle to know what to do with them. They describe effects but not cause because doctors don't fully understand the processes at work. When strangers in the street ask me 'what happened?' and gesture at *all of me*, I never know what to say. Where would I begin? None of the descriptions offer much explanation or support and some carry heavy stigma. Some therapies and medications seem to work for a while; others make it all much, much worse, so it's not easy to talk about those either. Any talk of cures is a matter of guesswork and luck and how patient and willing your doctor is to help you. That's often a matter of luck too.

For the most part, I must manage things on my own. I do everything I can to keep my mind healthy and helpful. I try to see clearly. I focus hard on the things I can control, however small; I focus on the world around me, on living and living and living. I make a good, rich life; I avoid questions; I let go of the rest. What else is there to do?

It doesn't matter here, in any case. This is not a book about the true nature of those names, whether they're 'real' illnesses, as some have long contested, which of them I have or don't have, or why I have them in the first place. It is simply about the life I have lived through all of it, and about the life I live now.

The miracle is, perhaps, that I am still here – that I continue – and that despite all that's come before, I believe my life to be good. That is the truth hidden under all of this: that I am deeply happy to be alive.

Usually, when you are unwell, people expect one of two stories: either you get better – you *beat it* – or you get worse and die. Stories of everyday living and undramatic, sustained existence, stories that don't end with cures or tragic climaxes but that are made up of slow, persistent continuation as you learn and change – stories about what happens *then* – they may be harder to tell, but I believe they're important too. I believe we need to tell more of them.

That is why this year I decided to be brave. I decided I would try to find a way to tell my story, to pin it down and spread it out in front of other people – in front of you – so we could look at it together. On the first of January, I made a resolution to try and write down my confused and searching past and the quiet days of my present, simply, honestly, and ignore the voice inside me that continues to tell me it is a worthless, unimportant story to tell. I have barely told a soul of it before. It was always too much to explain. I was always too complicated and I have felt too flawed and vulnerable in complexity's jumble. My life has made it easy to hide, and so I have, but I don't want to be something small and hidden any more. Mine is only one ordinary human life amongst countless, similar others, but it is a life that doesn't leave anything out: not grief, not pain, not delight, failure, confusion, nor joy. It holds and embraces all of it equally, and that, I have learnt, is nothing ordinary at all.

Here then are two stories: a slow life and a slow year, entwined. I give both to you, along with any hope and meaning you can glean from them.

Take my hand and walk with me, through my year, through my life. Let's see if we are the same at the end of it.

Josie George, 2018

Winter

I went to bed early last night. I shut the curtains on the last day of December but lay awake listening to the fireworks anyway, feeling a little lost. I wondered if they would wake my son. I secretly hoped they might so he would climb into my bed; so I could gather him in and say 'Happy New Year, my love' into his sweaty hair. I say it with the new morning instead as he wanders down the hallway, creased and sleepy. He stops still to say it back, grandly, earnestly, a messenger in my doorway: 'Happy New Year, Mummy.' I feel better then, knowing we've begun. Now he watches television in the front room and I make tea. It is still early. I think about the fireworks that I didn't see.

Slowly, unthinking, I begin to twist a teaspoon under the stutter of the cold tap, the old pipes only just resisting freezing, to make a firework of my own. I watch the light of the water turn and stumble and notice that its reflection makes a star in the upturned glass in the sink. The metal of the drying rack catches another. I imagine a whizz, a bang. I let my gaze follow, one spot of light to the next, and I know that this will be today's obsession – a way of moving through this first day of the year, a day that always feels odd, when I will wonder again who I am. A look down at my numb hands and my fingernails turn to mirror balls. I have to stop myself from playing the air like a pianist as I sit on the stool in the kitchen and wait for the toast to pop, my son's laughter drifting through the house, stopping then starting again. All morning, I do it – as I dress, as I rest again, holding onto the furniture as I go. I find willing lines of light along edges, in leather and wood, squinting my eyes to make them flare: my secret firework show.

Later, my dad arrives to collect us for a long overdue lunch together. He announces himself loudly: 'Here's Grumps!' – the teasing nickname we decided upon when my son was born. He asks if I'm OK, thinking that my frowning stare must mean something is wrong. I would never confess what I've been doing all morning, so I keep trying to smooth myself into reassurance and warm attention as he talks non-stop in the car the full eighteen miles to the house he shares with my stepmother, his grandson absent in his headphones on the back seat. I try to keep my eyes on my lap so I won't get distracted. I notice the skin around my dad's thumbs on the steering wheel has been bitten a familiar, ragged pink.

My dad booms about his step-children, about his prostate, about his Christmas on a cruise ship, his voice filling the car. His words fade as my eyes rove again. I can't help it now. A girl runs a pedestrian crossing in white trainers, her face hidden by an oversized scarf as her soles make sparks on the pavement. A thousand more lights shift in the beech hedge that runs alongside the main road. It is still clutching its bronze, dead leaves.

We pull up. We step inside. The dark house makes it easier to stop and be present with my family – I will not see them or much of anyone else again for a while – but later, when lunch and the blurred interactions are over, I sit back again in the car on our way home in the freezing, inky, evening rain, greedy for more, and nearly lose my mind at the sudden colour. No longer simply white light now, but red and green and blue. Lorry lights make wet Roman candles that bleed into the tarmac. There is light in the salt and light in the spray.

The true gift of it comes only as I finally close my eyes, exhausted, throbbing, buried deep in my bed again against the winter chill. I find every moment of light caught behind my eyelids. They flicker back into being, soft and enduring in the dark, to make a private night sky.

I fall asleep under stars.

I need you to trust me: this is a good way to start the year.

★

THEN

My childhood memories are of being at sea. My bedroom had begun as a garage before it was converted into a tatty, make-do playroom, but soon all the toys were moved out and it became my father's study. The old brown couch we had loved to jump on was suddenly, agonisingly forbidden. The door closed and required knocking. I had let the room go as a lost cause, until one weekend the couch, sharp with springs, was heaved into a skip and taken off to the tip with regret, the typewriter carried up to the box room where I had been sleeping, and I was told the big room was mine.

The walls were wide and newly white, the roof thin and flat, and soon I began to love the nights when it rained most of all. I asked for sheer fabric to hang over my bed in a canopy, sewing the crooked hems myself, and the inverted V shape from the ceiling hook made my bed look like a sailing boat. And there I lay for long hours, happy, awake, confused, wondering at the storm in my legs.

'Growing pains', we'd call them. Flashes of worry would flicker over my mother's face as she said that, like shadows through a train window. She was the same age I am now, my father a little older, and I was my son's age, perhaps a little younger: no more than eight, nine. Already I was a person with a story, a history – a *before* – and yet when I think about the beginning, I can't help but think of the boat.

'Where does it hurt, love?'

I'd try and gesture, running hands from my knees to my toes.

'Here,' I'd say. 'Deep inside. Like it's right in my bones.'

★

'Is it broken?' says a man, nodding to my mobility scooter while keeping cold hands in his pockets. He has a face like a scrubbed potato, his cheeks purple. The rest of him is all shoulders and shadow.

'Oh, no, thank you! I had just stopped to take photos of the puddles,' I say, and wave my camera. He nods again with a frown and gets into his car. It was school again this morning, for the first time after the Christmas holidays, and that means back to our routine. I make my way home from the playground and feel the sudden absence of my son like a hole in the air.

'Did you drop something?' a young woman asks a little farther down the road as I lean again over the pavement. The baby she holds is trying to gain purchase on his small hat, stretching with thick bricks of mittened hands but barely able to lift his arms in the snowsuit. It is covered in winged dragons.

'No, I . . . sorry . . . no, I'm fine. I was just looking at the ice on the puddles,' I try to say back over the angry wail that comes from somewhere inside the swollen polyester shape bouncing on her angled hip, but the woman just smiles briefly and, still looking at me, carries on a conversation with her friend. I turn the corner until they are out of sight and then I stop again.

'What are you doing?' a third voice says, dark laced boots drawing closer to my bent head. I look up and she's tall and sharp with the kind of tight mouth that waits in readiness to be appalled.

'I was just taking photos. There's lots of ice today,' I say, smiling.

'Oh! I see. Good for you. These roads are dreadful, aren't they? I've always thought someone should do something about them. Such a state.'

'That's not what I meant,' I return, too late as she strides past me, neck long. Her pace doesn't slow as her heel splinters another puddle with a crunch.

I wait a while for the coast to clear and then I grin, devilish, and make my way over to look at that one too.

★

THEN

Spoons full of sickly Calpol were dispensed on the nights when my uncomfortable restlessness led me to cross the narrow hallway. I'd stand blinking and miserable at the gap in the sitting-room door. My parents would look up from their separate armchairs: my mother with the frown line that always bisected her forehead, just above her nose, my father still in his workday shirt but without his tie, his chest thin, his hair thinner, a paper spread out on his lap. I believe that's how it went. I remember Mum guiding me back and sitting at the end of my bed under the canopy, gently talking me through a relaxation exercise that started at my head and ended at my feet, her voice soft. 'That's it. Just breathe in, nice and slow. Now a long breath out.' She breathed with me.

I'd feel the warm energy of my attention move around my body. I was always good at that: good at following instructions. Go to sleep, arms. Go to sleep, back. Go to sleep, legs. It was like a game. By the end, when she would tiptoe out, her quiet exhale lingering after her, I'd be still and serene in the shared relief of it. I didn't like to interrupt the finality of the moment to tell her that the pain hadn't gone, so I'd just try and float on it, like flotsam, until slowly, slowly, sleep would come, long after the line of light around my half open bedroom door had gone out.

I kept that bed for over twenty years, sat by it with my own restless child. I put a canopy over it for him too, but it was red this time, and I made a skull-and-crossbones flag to ride its point in warning. Perhaps I thought it would make it a safer ride.

The white boat wasn't the first bed I remember though: there were others. I remember bawling at the orange light that hung from the ceiling of my first bedroom in our first house when I was two, maybe three, the room cast in its pallid, dead sun glow. I remember my mother bobbing in the single bed across the room from me, trying to sleep, exhausted. That house was tall and dark and the rooms stank of Marmite and beer from the twin factories at the bottom of the busy main road. When I was four, a decision was made to move us twenty miles away, from East Midlands to West, to the square house with the garage in the town I still live in today, to escape the smell and maybe, I think, something else – some unspoken unhappiness – but we, I, never went further than that. The new house sat on a nicer, nondescript housing estate right by the motorway. We swapped the smell for the noise and agreed it was a better deal. I always liked the sound of that motorway. I thought it sounded like waves on a shore.

They tell me that I was bright and wilful and a happy child but rarely comfortable. Colic spasmed through my thin body long past the age it was supposed to, and when I fell or hurt myself, I'd be impossible to soothe for hours, shaking with the intensity of it. Even before we moved, I had begun to be passed around paediatricians in a rhythm of appointments. As I grew, there were special diets, particular plates of food at my friends' birthday parties that I learnt to shake my head at politely, endless sheets of paper carrying stars and faces designed to chart my ailing digestion, my sporadic sleeping, my struggling bladder control. I remember standing by the coat pegs when I was maybe seven years old, alone after yet another trip to the toilet, clutching my grid of smiling and sad faces, and realising with a sudden, blushing horror that these sheets were something shameful. I mustn't let anyone see them. I kept my spare knickers hidden in the bottom of my school bag.

These moments are rare in my memory though. Mostly, I remember being free and at peace. I remember being a rosy-cheeked angel with a tinsel halo singing 'Away in a Manger' at the top of my lungs at my first school Nativity play. I remember Sundays spent sat on a dusty floor, using the hard pew like a desk and drawing pictures as my father's voice filled the church, wincing as a pen rolled off and clattered on the floor during prayers. I remember holding hands with my friend Natalie when we were five and watching in open-mouthed, adoring awe as her mum checked her blood sugar, the round pearl of blood on Natalie's finger the most beautiful, horrifying thing I had ever seen. I remember carefully writing on the blue lines of my schoolbooks, my chest aching with pride with each new book and each new year.

★

We are settling back into it now, him and me. School. Work. Homework. Chores. I try to write. I try to keep the house clean. I try to make us things to eat that don't make me feel too ashamed. It is still so cold. We wear hats and gloves and scarves to go to school and I do not take them off when I get home.

The door knocks twice today. A sign on my window says, 'Please Be Patient'. The first time it is a food delivery I had forgotten about. I never manage to order the right things so there is already a list on the whiteboard of essentials that I've forgotten. My son writes things up there to help too: P.E. KIT ON WEDNESDAYS. CHESS CLUB ON THURSDAYS. I LOVE YOU MUMMY. The second time, it is a woman with a clipboard and my medication: painkillers, anti-spasmodics, beta-blockers. They just send them now, so there's no need to take up an appointment.

The cold air fills the house each time I open the door, but I still spend a while looking out before I close it again, letting my breath puff out like a great, slow engine. I hold onto the cupboard to look at the dark, enduring green of the conifers and the brown, dead tangle of the wild rose in my neighbour's garden on the opposite corner, where the wrens hide in winter and split the sky with their song. The man who lives there is the only one here with a grassy front yard and a drive. The wall that surrounds it makes a noticeably stark barrier in contrast to our front doors that tumble straight out onto the pavement. I don't know whether he chose the house for the grass and the wall, or if the grass and the wall changed him, but he doesn't speak to us, in any case. As I stand and look, he eyes me from the car with the motor running, full of suspicion. He keeps his upstairs curtains closed and the paint is peeling off the house, bright blue under cream.

My phone tells me that it has been exactly three years since I took a wrong path. It was a rare January, one when my legs let me roam occasionally, and I ended up climbing to the top of a high hill. It felt like a mountain. I remember that the summit grass cracked as I sat on it and that I had three apples in my bag; I ate two and fed the cores to the wild mountain ponies who joined me. It was one of the most wildly romantic things I have ever done and I didn't care that it was going to hurt. Three years ago, I sat alone on the cold ground of the Long Mynd and felt my heart as if it were held in cupped hands and raised up to the sky.

My range on foot now is about eight metres. My feet often drag and must be pulled along one at a time. The world around me shifts and lurches, turning my movement into a forward clamber that requires both hands. It is agonisingly slow, to experience and to watch, but I get there in the end. Then I must rest for a good long time.

You'd think someone who has always found movement difficult would have finally evolved to be a sedentary, restful creature, happy to circle the nest, but I haven't. I'm still a wanderer, right the way through to my middle. I spend all day testing the edges of my tether just in case it has stretched a little again because you never know and I am not afraid. Sometimes I bundle myself up with a cardigan over my jumper and a coat over that and I walk the short backyard path up and down, sitting on a hard chair by the gate until I'm ready to go again. Most of the time, I just walk around the house, or walk to the door and open it and look. Walk and rest, walk and rest, a few steps at a time. Some days, I get so angry, I want to throw my life at the wall, but I have learnt to breathe through that and walk and rest some more. I do it over and over until I've filled a day. If I could unhook my body from my will, I would cover leagues within minutes, but I can't, and so all the energy must find another way out.

It manifests these days as a quiet intensity. My gaze has intensified as my body has slowed. Now, I notice everything, and I am hungry for everything: hungry to experience every detail I can. I make sure I don't overlook a thing. If eight metres is my limit, I will know it better than anyone else on this earth. I study my surroundings as if they were an encyclopaedia.

Today, the walk back to the kitchen leaves my pulse as wild as it was through that climb into Shropshire's clouds. I sit and admire the view just the same until it settles again. Our black cat is sitting on the windowsill. I let myself climb the dip and peak of his fur, feeling just as cold, just as nipped around my edges as that left-behind January day, and there, there again, something in me soars.

Much of the nature writing and poetry I read talks of connecting to yourself and to the land by walking, exploring, by rediscovering wildness. But what if you can't walk and can't leave, what then? What if your wildness is dead roses and walled yards, mossy rooftops and cold neighbours?

There are some who would scoff that my cat's back doesn't count as a mountain, but who are they to say? Today, I climbed it in the winter air all the same. The same you visits each place, whether it is a cat or a mountain, or the bin-strewn ginnel that runs behind the terraces and that erupts with bright bluebells in the spring. What you bring with you can be nothing or everything. You can leave with as little or as much.

There are days when I can't help but feel such envy. There are days when I watch the world go about its activities, through the windows of my house and the screen of my phone and the open door of my front room, my neighbours pulling away in their cars, and I burn with longing. 'Oh, all the things they must see!' I think. But even then, a voice inside of me whispers back, in challenge, in defiance, 'Ah, but Jo. Think of all the things they must miss.'

★

THEN

My brother was born two years after me, but that moment of beginning is long forgotten. He appears in my memory as a fidgety pre-schooler, his glasses like huge, round moons on his small face. I remember his toothy smile, his constant chatter drifting down the stairs even when he was entirely alone. I remember looking around the door of his bedroom and seeing him address an army of jumble-sale teddies with confident authority. It would make my mum wince when he bought them with his sweatily-held ten pence pieces, their grubby stuffing spilling out onto the floor of the church hall, but they were precious for some vital reason so she'd let him bring them home anyway and patch them up until they took up more space in his bed than he did. I remember lining up my own collection of My Little Ponies on the white gloss windowsill of the box room I slept in back then, before I moved downstairs. It swam with condensation in the morning and left their pony feet and pony tails soaking. They too had arrived one by one thanks to my own hoarded ten pences.

I remember feeling safe and loved and part of something, and although I did not know then what a gift that was, I do now.

★

It is the weekend and my son is home. Every other weekend, he stays fifteen miles away with his father, but not this one; this weekend is mine.

My ex-husband is kind. On the days he does arrive to pick up our boy and his bag of carefully packed clothes, he smiles and nods and exchanges news but doesn't look directly at me. I often want to tell him that I love him, does he know that? I love him like a second brother. I want to reach and put a hand on his arm as I say it, but the words are hard to say and I know they might be painful to hear, after everything that once happened between us, so I don't say them, and I keep my hands in my lap. I have lost the right to touch. I just smile and nod right back.

The door closing with my son on the other side of it always leaves me shaken. Without the routine of school or him to ground me, I often drift, unsure of what to do. Some weekends when he's away, I forget to eat, to phone anyone, or I end up working too hard for too long until I'm sick. Other weekends, the freedom of it is a new dawn and I clutch at the uninterrupted, demand-free time like a life raft, grinning at the silence, at my writing, my books, at anything and everything, until the Sunday afternoon when suddenly I start to miss his small, angular body more than I can bear and can do nothing but stare down the remaining hours until he's home again.

I'm glad he's here with me today even though we can't really leave the house. Even though I worry, often, that I'm boring.

It feels like it's always been just the two of us. It hasn't, of course. When his dad stands in the front room, it is an echo of an earlier, forgotten time when this was his space too, but the eight years since he moved out is most of our son's life and in many respects, it's been most of my mine too. Before feels like shadows. Sometimes I think we were born at the same time, my son and I: both of us together. We have grown quietly alongside one another.

I do not know what is nature and what is nurture but my son has always been a happy yet subdued child, never wanting to wander far. He didn't figure out how to make his speech sounds come together in the right way until he was five and although since then there have been days of long chatter, it is still usually of the earnest kind that comes only after thought: 'People think pigeons are boring but they have two sets of eyelids so that's wrong.

Good morning, Mummy.' His serious statements are interspersed with sudden laughter that lights him up as though you've blown oxygen right through him and it is all the more special for the fact it's hard won. He swings between sudden, unshakeable belief and inventive, sceptical dismissal, and nothing you say can convince him otherwise.

His energy comes out with focus and passion. He gets his fire from things that align and provide safe, solid worlds to walk in – through order and rightness and familiar rules and systems. I get mine by pulling everything apart to touch what's inside, driven to understand and in the process, discover whole new worlds. When his day stumbles, he dissolves in loud, sudden panic, his body and his mind making a kind of firework. He marvels at my calm and thinks it some kind of magic. He has a freckle on his top lip that makes me ache.

He spends a lot of time lost in thought, in music, film and games, and he has a gentleness and patience in his way with other people that makes my breath catch. The way he talks to our cat when he thinks no one is listening would tell you everything you need to know about how much heart runs through him: 'You are the best cat,' he'll whisper, 'and I love you even though you bite me sometimes and don't like cuddling. Are you having a good day? I think you are.'

He is my devoted, frowning, careful professor. My contrast. My childish rebellions make him shake his head at me: 'Muum.' Whereas I am often enamoured by the world, he is suspicious of it, and there is conflict in that at times, in his rigid, unbending certainty and in my silly, forgetful abstraction, but we do OK. He brings a steady hand and I bring wide eyes.

And through all that, we make a life. We talk a lot, but we spend even more time saying nothing at all in a way that is warm and close, each often lost in something different, side by side. Like me, he is drawn to touch and even now, grown tall, will keep orbiting back to wrap arms around my waist, to push forehead against my cheek, and stay like that awhile.

We are most ourselves on Sundays, our most quiet and absorbed and our most loving.

Today, the first snow falls. I let it coat my dressing gown as I blunder around the garden with my camera, ignoring the cold, and he watches me through the window with an old smile.

★

THEN

Before I moved downstairs to the room with the bed like a sailing boat, I used to sit on the top step of the stairs at night and listen to the deadened sounds of my parents watching television. I could never make out many individual words and I preferred it that way. When the odd word managed to escape through the closed sitting-room door to find me, it only felt more important for its sudden clarity. I'd sit patiently in the dark and see what came. The distant, precipitant crescendo of a TV show's theme tune; the hum of the fridge changing gears; the scrape and clunk as my mother laid the iron to rest; my Dad's solitary cough resonant. I'd hold my breath as they moved around, count down how long it took for the kettle to boil as they made a drink before they went to bed, knowing I was running out of time before I'd be discovered. It all felt sacred, like a promise.

I remember the feel of the carpet beneath my bare feet and the yellow streetlamp cutting a stripe across my toes from the gap in the curtains. I remember that secret vigil; that ceremony of determined, self-created hope. I remember all the times since that I've stopped and looked inside myself, as though lifting the bonnet of a car. I've always found it. Hope has always been like the beating of my heart: as constant, as reliable, and as easily forgotten.

How easy it would have been to sit in my bed, chest tight, waiting for meaning to arrive like a switched-on light. Even then, I seemed to know that it didn't work like that.

I was maybe six years old then, before things got bad.

★

There is little of interest to say today. I mostly sleep and drift, and smile at the twin points of my cat's ears protruding from behind a roll of the duvet. My mum, who lives across town, offered to do the school runs to save us from a January soaking. The rain makes long lines down the dirty windows. All my energy goes into slow trips back and forth to the toilet.

I am embarrassed by my mundanity. You'd think it would be the easiest thing in the world to write about my days but I don't find it easy because I want to tell the truth. I wish my truth was pretty but it's not.

We're told that it is beauty, success and excitement that make us lovable. These are the things that will save us. Filter and tweak our bodies and our lives until only what's pleasing, impressive or entertaining remains and the right people and opportunities will be drawn to us.

The most painful thing is that it's true, or at least it seems to be. We've all of us lived long enough to see what's rewarded. We've all of us lived long enough to see what repels. What's worse is that we see everyone around us doing the same – we watch what they choose, for themselves and for others. We watch who is chosen. It only makes us believe it all a little more. It makes vulnerability risky. It makes my vulnerability feel terrifying.

Today I remember that writing out my days means making a choice: either I share the truth, or I try to twist and tidy. Here, there's only me, my scattered memories, this tiny, jumbled house I struggle to leave, a handful of dingy, dirty streets in the rain. We fill the whole frame. To put on a show with my memories instead is tempting. I know I could do that. The telling of memories can so easily become a clever sleight of hand. We can dazzle or shock with our recollections to make people look away from who we really are now.

I recognise this feeling of wanting to hide, this temptation. I've felt this before. I haven't lived with another adult since my ex-husband moved out, and although there is loneliness in that at times, the invisibility can be addictive. I am not often seen, and that can be a sly, convenient place to deceive from. It makes it all too easy to arrange a life where you only show the things you think are lovable and easy. You can quickly curate an identity you feel is more pleasing, special. The lure of social media makes it especially tempting. If I want company, I can have it with a press of my phone. You could make *these* people like you, says a voice, if you play it right; if you don't say too much.

It took real intimacy to break this in me. When I got to know my best friend Jude, four, five years ago, and realised that she only lives three streets away from me, I lost the ability to hide too much or too often.

'Oi!' she'd call from the other side of the road as we passed on the morning school run. 'Fancy a fried egg sandwich and a cuppa at mine in a bit? We can even use the fancy mugs.'

My friendships had all been distant or sporadic before. I have always existed well alongside people but have rarely known how to overlap. With her, it was different, right from the start, and soon I found myself up against the choice at the heart of it all: was I going to be careful? Was I only going to say and share and let her see the things that I thought would make her like me, or was I going to show her the truth? For me, exhaustion made the battle shorter and so, soon, there I was, whole and raw, hoping I wouldn't make her run away. 'As if I would, you knob,' she said, when I admitted it. 'You're stuck with me, I'm afraid.'

Fear makes us silent and much that is valuable can be lost in silence. I'm trying to remember that again now; to resist the temptation to fall into it just because I'm afraid to be seen. The world has told me every single day that I am lesser in some way, but I don't help by believing it.

Either I believe that illness, pain, and our naturally chaotic minds are something undesirable and shameful to be hidden away, and so hide myself in response, or I don't believe that. And if I don't, and oh god, I don't, then I'm going to have to start being braver with my visibility and braver with my truth.

Either I believe that love is something shallow and narrow, something that only really responds to perfection and beauty, that requires you to be *special*, or I believe love is something bigger than that. And if I believe it is something bigger, and oh god, I do, then I'm going to have to start giving people the chance to see me as I really am, and how I really was, too.

My phone buzzes. It's Jude. 'Hey, lovely. I missed you this morning. How's today going?'

Sometimes, people don't run, I know that now. That is what true love is. That is the terror and joy of intimacy.

★

THEN

Was I seven when it all changed? Eight? These early memories slip and slide. I do not remember when I started to get so tired, only that after years of hardly ever sleeping, suddenly sleep seemed to be all I could do.

I recall little of its substance. I remember being so exhausted that to sit unsupported or even to be upright was to feel like something was draining from me, like blood, like the blood on Natalie's finger, like sand through the funnel on the school sand table. I remember whole days when sounds felt strange, like they were either too loud or very far away. I'd lie in the middle of it and wonder why I couldn't touch it.

'Josie's had her plug pulled out again', my parents would say, and we'd laugh with the kind of laughter that aches, not knowing what else to do.

So began long sofa days. I would often retreat into my head and stay there. There was nothing else to do. Outside, everything hurt and everyone frowned and asked me questions that made me feel small and ashamed. 'Maybe you're worried about something?', the GP would say as I sat pale and crumpled in the consulting chair. 'Do you like school?'

Of course I liked school, I'd say, surprised. I loved school! I was good at school and I loved project work especially. A new topic was announced every half term and we'd get to keep our work in brand-new card folders that made my skin prickle with pleasure. I'd turn mine into works of art, into proper books with ANCIENT EGYPT and HABITATS and TRANSPORT written in beautiful lettering on the cover. The ones that were thin, from when I had missed too many days, frustrated me. I begged to be allowed to work on them at home, using books from the tattered library near the papershop to copy facts and pictures carefully onto lesson sheets of my own devising, at least for an hour or two before the wooze of it all pulled me back to the sofa.

Being busy made me happy, happier than anything, and if I couldn't be busy out there, I would just be busy in my head. That's what I decided.

Books. More, please – I had work to do. I devoured them by the carrier-bag-full in long pulls between frequent sleeps. My favourite teacher would appear at the door of our house some evenings to restock me, her voice gravelly from decades of cigarettes, her blonde hair ashy and thin, as if a part of her was burning, all the time. 'I think you'd like this one,' she'd say, with a twinkle. She'd pull them from her own shelves, somehow understanding my urgent need. I'd want her to come in, to stay, but she never did. She lived with a man that no one approved of and then later ran away to Germany, or so I heard. For the time I knew her, I loved her more than I knew how to say. Thanks to her, I played secret gardens with Colin and Dickon, explored midnight worlds with Tom. I watched the snow fall from my chalet school window, roamed an island with Gilbert, tamed dragons, shrunk myself to an inch high and lived a life under the grandfather clock. I would not be stopped. I would not be still.

I knew exactly who I was and to think back is to remember a blaze of fierceness in my chest that makes me burn again with fondness. I pulsed with life. It bubbled in me; it just couldn't get out. Ideas filled me like new hearts, pumping, pumping. I was real! I was alive! I was sure of it; it was just the rest of the world that was out of reach. I was so tired. Why couldn't I touch the things around me? There was a wall between me and everything I loved, but it was still there, I'd tell myself, trying to calm the silent panic, it was OK. School, my teacher, my bike – they were all still there.

I'd close my eyes and listen to the gentle click of the cricket ball on the television, the low burble of commentary like water, picturing the tanned curve of Dad's knees in his weekend shorts as he sat in the armchair across the room. 'Howzat!' he'd cry, and, with that, all would be well again.

★

I thought I'd try to get out again today. I haven't been to our community centre in a while. The net curtain twitches as I navigate the narrow path through the sheltered housing complex to get to it. My most attentive neighbour has heard me coming again: the hum and rattle of the scooter. I think she must listen out.

She stands at the window of her ground-floor flat, her left arm in a blue sling, her wrinkled face framed by a halo of soft white. This is our ritual, always the same, every time I pass. She smiles a soft, sad smile and waves with her good arm just a little. I know she gets confused sometimes, that she worries for me, so I always give a bit of extra gusto as I wave back, craning my neck so my scarf doesn't hide my mouth or its reassuring smile. I know I look younger and

more vulnerable than I am. 'Look, see, I'm fine!' I try
to say, even though I don't feel it really, not today.

Difference is an odd thing. I'm beginning to realise
that it's a spectrum — no, a wedge. Yes, that's it. We all
have a place in it, we're all different, but some of us are
undeniably more different than others.

The thin edge of the wedge is a strange place to
exist. The further down into difference you go, the
more of you that doesn't match, the tighter it all gets.
Fewer and fewer people look like you or act like you
or live like you. Fewer and fewer environments fit your
body or meet your needs, spaces catered for the masses.
Opportunities and choices shrink. It gets harder to
see yourself in other people, harder to find common
ground. You begin to realise what a privilege it is to
have the ability to blend in, and what it really means
when you don't, can't. More and more people begin
either to look past you and through you, or to stare.
I have never decided which is worse. I suspect getting
older feels the same: I've just had to learn it sooner.

Through the gate and over the bump. I tip my head
back to greet the trees because I've missed them. Two
larches like arrows, needles spent now, their winter
shapes stark, and a blue cedar like a fuzzy bear. That
one doesn't mind the cold. The frost outlines the clover
on the grass that forms a circle in front of the centre
itself. I know from memory that this tree is elder, this
one ash, and over there run young hornbeams all in

a line, although each of those is anonymous now, no leaf growth yet to give them away. Some days, when I come here, all I do is sit by the window and relish that there are so many trees in one place because that is rare around here.

Three years ago, the community centre opened a hundred metres from my house. Around that time I had taken another tumble, deeper down into that wedge of difference. I was trying to learn what that meant for me and how to navigate it when Jude told me this place had opened between our houses. Two minutes from my front door was about the limit of my independence and I will thank the stars until I die that fate aligned us like that, my community centre and me, because I could get to it. Suddenly, I could get *somewhere*. Somewhere was better than anything I'd had in a while.

As I drive through the automatic doors, I can hear Tina laughing in the kitchen. She manages the small army of matronly hens who fuss and flap and cackle as they make you your cheap coffee and who swear when they don't think you're listening. Tina undercharges me for my food and slips me pieces of cake that need eating up. I love her and all of them as family. They each call a greeting as they see me, waking Frank who is nodding over his omelette. My friend Neil calls a booming 'HIYA!' from his seat at the computer desks. He is looking at pictures of theme parks: his favourite.

The community centre is modern, wide and spacious, the ceiling high. The windows face south and so even if I do nothing else today, I know the short day's light will move in long waves across the tables, chairs, sofas and armchairs, casting great, slow, shadows.

I come here whenever I can, even if it's just for an hour or two. I come here for the free warmth when it's cold like today because I can never get my house to feel warm. I come for the internet and high-backed seats that support my head if I need them, and the armchairs that have just enough room for you to tuck your feet underneath you, if you slip your shoes off. I come here for a toilet that doesn't require a climb up steep stairs, and for food and drink placed into my hands by people who know my face instead of getting to 3 p.m. only to realise that I haven't eaten a thing. I come here because there is nowhere else that I can bloody well get to by myself, but above all else, I come here to stop being different for a while, for my community centre is a temple of difference, and it is more special in that than it knows.

Here, everyone is different, or at least us regulars are. The centre adjoins a mass of assisted-living flats, a health centre, a dementia care home and a women's refuge, and houses its own classrooms for people with complex learning needs. There are meeting rooms for businesses and a dance and yoga studio, but their tidy, energetic visitors are the ones who stand out here, not us.

Some of us talk too loudly, using our bodies and our sounds in different ways. Like Neil; like Joanne who weaves her body back and forth in a distinctive pattern of rocking. Others, like red-haired, smiling Louise, don't speak at all. No two bodies look alike and no two faces. Some of us have always been different, others have been made different by age. I, with my odd, lurching gait, get to join a cheerful legion of shufflers and hunched backs and sagging skin. At any time of count, at least three people will be asleep. Today there is Frank, and wizened Henry in the corner in his hi-vis jacket. Lucy sits with her coat on, clutching her handbag, weeping as she often does, waiting for the community transport that will take her to the local day centre. She has forgotten to put her teeth in again, but I have got used to that and can now translate and soothe the day's small distresses from her incoherent mumbles until she settles. She's only fifty-nine but she's had a hard, hard life. I've slowly translated that from each day's mumbles too, as she's told me her story, little by little.

This place is the best and brightest, safest place I know. Places like this are rare and precious. They split that narrow end of the wedge wide open. Places like this let all of us breathe.

I settle into my usual place and pull out my notebook and my fountain pen, full to the brim today, unexpectedly, with a grief for it all. And with legs that couldn't manage even two steps together to get from my scooter to the chair, nobody stares, and nobody minds.

'Here, duck. Let me get you a coffee.'

★

THEN

My parents both worked, my mum as a social worker, my dad for the church. Mum couldn't always take the extra time off when I started to get sick and then Dad got sick too. 'It's a kind of illness that happens in your head,' my mum explained to my younger brother and me when we asked where our dad had gone. 'It makes him feel very sad.'

At eight years old, I couldn't imagine how *my* dad, who constantly told jokes and filled any room he stood in, I couldn't understand how *he* could be sad. I couldn't imagine feeling sad enough that you would need to be in a hospital. It alarmed me; I didn't know sadness could do that. But when we visited, I don't remember being afraid, only thinking it funny that Dad, a man of shirts and ties, was in his familiar brown felted dressing gown and slippers in the middle of the day. He walked around and joked as he always did, there in the strange rooms full of chairs and dazed, lumbering people, so I knew it couldn't be too bad. And, besides, it wasn't long before he was home and out of the door in his cheap blue suits after breakfast again, so I soon forgot about this dangerous sadness.

We'd have to make sure to tidy up before he came home for tea and there, he'd perform the skits and lines I knew off by heart as we sat in a small square around our dining table. I'd grin and grin and swing my sore legs and roll my eyes at my brother who solemnly, silently, over-chewed his meat until he had to spit it out in slimy grey globules. My mother would calmly ignore this charade for long weeks until it landed on a day when something invisible had been stretched taught enough, when she'd finally interrupt Dad's performance to say, exasperated, 'Oh, just SWALLOW it,' pushing back her chair to fetch more water. It was rare to see her lose her temper and she was always pink a long time after. I remember the flush of her beneath the tight, mousey perm that she got sick of and later grew into a respectably long bob, coarse with bleach, only to hate that secretly too. I'd primly empty my plate afterwards, languishing in knowing that *I* was good, at least, still believing that all was right with the world. Dad would slip away soon after, to a church meeting or back to the typewriter to work on the dense, questioning books of theology he wrote, while we were ushered up for baths. Mum would apologise for getting cross. And all proceeded just as it always did for the two months or more that it took for me to get sick again.

★

It is my birthday today. I look in the mirror and conclude that I look just the same, but then I always think that. Later, Jude will pick me up in the car and I will get to lie on her sofa. She will bring me easy food and cups of tea and take the piss out of me in the very best way. 'Race you,' she'll grin as I lumber and laugh my way down the hallway to find she has prepared a spot by the window, with something just right to rest my feet on. There, we will blather like sprites about her longings and plans and my uneventful days, and it won't matter if I fall asleep when we put a film on. 'I'm sorry I didn't want to do anything more exciting today,' I'll say, inevitably, and she will reply that she doesn't need exciting and that, to be honest, she's knackered too and this is just what she needed. She'll jump from clown to expressive, tender-heart in a moment: 'I love you for a hundred reasons, but one of them is that you make me and everyone else feel better about going slowly too.'

I try to tidy things up before I leave. Things have a way of running away from me here – abandoned mugs, half-folded clothes – as I wait for a better day.

I have a habit of leaving flowers in vases long past their best, until they are puckered and wrinkled, losing their petals and manners. This habit's not from idleness or fatigue though, this is more a kind of lived intention: I don't give up on things any more. I want to love beyond first bloom and easy convenience, all through the inevitable changing and fading. I want to see what happens when things stop being perfect.

I have learnt, painfully, that love without curiosity is short-lived. I want a life now where love doesn't run out; to see things for everything they are, for as long as they live. And so, I let my flowers turn every colour they know, change their shape, cast new shadows, in defiance and in pride. Perhaps, I think, if I do, I will learn how to love my people better. Myself, even.

A friend had sent me roses the week before. Now, as I pick their rasping, fading blooms out of the withered, dank foliage to keep what I can a little longer, a birthday card lands on the doormat and it is only then that I feel it: I feel the year move me on. I don't open it; I press it to my fevered face like cool hands. I have been sick again. The flu this time. It was bronchitis before that. There's always something.

My mother phones as I'm getting my coat on. I had just been thinking of her because her hands were always cold. As a child, I would take them and press them to my head on days like this. Can she pop in on her way back from work later? I look around at the mess and the dishes in the sink I'm about to abandon and cringe but say yes, yes, I'd love that. I can already picture her at the door, her familiar smile, her short posture at ease and a little lopsided. I always know it's her before she knocks; she walks in a clip-clop that I'd know anywhere. She's in her sixties now, her thick hair cropped and grey, comfortable at last. When I look at Mum, I see all her past years overlaid and I see her own mother too, who I loved. I see my past and my future.

I have never been afraid of getting older, perhaps because I know that the life I'm living now is good practice. Year on year, I am continually amazed and thankful that I get this chance to keep living; that the people I love keep on getting the chance to age around me. I find myself looking forward to seeing what my own next changing will look like, a slow fade or a bright riot, what crisping and sloughing and new blush I have waiting.

I think it could be beautiful, but if not, then maybe interesting would do.

★

THEN

Each day I was sick, a list was worked through, of friends and childminders and other neighbourhood mums. I would sit on the stairs and watch my mother's forehead to gauge her concern and consternation as she made the early-morning calls. I'd feel the guilt of it rise hot in me, like a second fever, as I waited to hear who I would be taken to. I had my favourites, of course, and the names that would make my heart drop like a pebble, small and unheard.

Gwen's house came with flowers and with Sweep, an old English sheepdog puppy who had to have the hair cut from his face to stop him running into the furniture. He'd be kept apart, to let me rest, but I'd hear his whines from the childgate at the kitchen door and know I'd get to push my fingers through the mop of him later. I was happy about that. Gwen never made me feel like a nuisance, her soft, lilting voice only cheerful comfort, only delight. Her eyes would disappear entirely when she smiled: her smile took up so much of her.

Cerys had a round-faced, flamed-haired, freckled daughter, who warmed up the rooms she was in but who hissed and spat in a way that made me uncertain, so I was always relieved to know that she'd be at school when I was there. Cerys was gentler and all freckle too and would stand to make round, buttery Welsh cakes on the stove top. They stuck to the roof of my mouth; I'd happily eat half a dozen, given the chance. Between turns of the cakes, she'd lay out a craft to do together on the dining table after lunch, if I was up to it. I'd try to will myself better so I could.

Asha's house meant welcome new scents and tastes and a rich cardamom smell to the sofa that I loved, all in a dark, silent house. Quiet, nodding, clever Asha would whisper into the echo of it and let me take books from her children's bookcases to read, encyclopaedias and textbooks that I devoured and used to make more pages for my project books, copying out the illustrations with unfamiliar pens. Her husband would appear at lunchtime sometimes. I always wanted to climb into his lap, wishing I could touch his neat turban. He shone with gentleness and I suspected him to be one of the best men in the world.

Linda's, on the other hand, was always cold. I felt lonelier there; long hours spent staring through the closed patio doors at a featureless lawn. In my memory, it is always raining. It was an especially long walk to the kitchen to ask for a drink, and to the bathroom, and I'd sit on the landing afterward, unseen, spent, assessing the angle of my descent.

Karen's came with a sense of my being in the way; of blinking, overwhelmed at the crowded fridge door that wheezed how busy everyone was. There were always people at the door, and a toddler who would pinch me and cry straight after to mask his crime, his eyes vicious, victorious. His sister was a bully too, cruel and jeering, and that, more than anything, was what would make me fall numb with betrayal when Mum mouthed this particular name at me through her telephone calls. This was the house of my enemy.

'Dear God. Please not Karen,' I would chant in a whisper, well-schooled in prayer, wondering if this counted.

★

Cabin fever has hit me like a tackle to the ribs. I don't know why. The morning gave me breakfast out at a new café with Jude and a movie reel of grey sky through her car window, but it isn't enough today. The community centre won't do. I can't breathe, I can't breathe even there. I need to get out of this house, away from these streets.

The mobility scooter helps on days like these, but my body's battery does not power as well as the scooter's does, so trips must still be kept short as I try not to slump over the handlebars. The scooter battery comes with its own problem too. Impossibly heavy, charging it means a brace and a painful heave, and so I can't do it all that often. I didn't charge it last night. I know that now it will be almost dead.

Four bars. Four bars of freedom and escape I could have had, but it had shown two yesterday, and once you get two you lose them faster. I know this as I pull on boots and coat and scarf in the near dark and shut the door anyway. I need out. Don't care.

I'll give it till it drops to one, that's what I'll do. I'll go as far as that takes me, and then I'll turn back and pray it lasts. And so I do, breathing hard to try and get some air in my lungs, huddled under the ridiculous, oversized blanket I've wrapped myself in to try and stave off the cold that brings me down more quickly than anything else. I steer away from traffic and industrial grey and towards the marshland that runs behind our housing estate. I can't get into it, its paths uneven and inaccessible, but a paved strip runs along the edge which means I can get close enough to at least see its sky. I head there: a slow, farcical runaway in a rainbow blanket and a bright blue hat.

The bar blinks out five minutes in, just as I begin to hit a wilder space and breathe a little easier, and I stop, dutifully, swearing loudly. There is no view to tell of – the fading light dulling everything, my low sightline blocked by winter hedges – but I sit and wait anyway, and watch, because I am nothing if not hopeful.

I am facing west, I realise, the early sunset hidden behind cloud except in one place. A tear in the air shaped like a long-necked bird in flight glows orange and I watch it burn and close. And perhaps it is the colour that tunes my eye because then I see more of it, through the hedge right in front of me.

There. A flash of orange and a singular bend of white that can only mean one thing in all the world and all of time.

A swan above and a swan below, I think, as I turn and drive back home. I smile, renewed.

I don't need much, that's the thing.

★

THEN

I do not remember company on any of my childhood sofa days. I do not remember conversation, apart from the odd, hesitant exchange. I mostly remember being very, very quiet, my socked toes stretching away from me like sails on a horizon. I felt transparent, like a ghost in a story, or a girl trapped in a distant wing of a house, out of time. Only my body, always so heavy, reminded me where I was.

I was feverish often, glands swelling like golf balls, and so the days passed in a blur of half-sleep and dropped books. I wondered what my friends were saying about me when I wasn't there or if they'd forgotten me entirely. A week would feel like a year and each would involve a shuffling of favours, the names changing day by day so that I didn't take up too much of anyone's time or patience.

Mum would pick me up after work, her cool hand pressed to my forehead appraisingly. 'You look better!' she'd say, optimistically, brightly, and I'd nod and smile to please her, even if I didn't feel it. She must have said those same words a thousand times in the three decades since: an inexhaustible statement of hope that maybe there wouldn't be a next time, this time. Maybe, maybe.

★

I guess I am in some trouble when I wake up. My movements come too slow or not at all as I try to pull on yesterday's jeans and jumper, in easy reach on my chair. The thrumming pain I feel is louder than usual. There is a sense of being compressed, of being squashed; a weight. I slide my way down the stairs in my tight lead suit, the cat by my side.

I begin the morning anyway. I do not like to assume what the day will be like, however it begins. I have it written on a card by my bed: 'Wait and see!' I am obedient and try to wait and see.

My son is away this weekend. I try to follow the steadying map of our routine without him, inch by inch. I sit to do the writing I have planned, each muscle around my pen coaxed forward, a dead weight, until like a wind-up doll at the end of her turn, I slowly come to a stop.

Feeling your own nervous system overload is a sensation I will never get used to. It seems to come when I've done too much, although what counts as 'much' may be laughable, unpredictable. I ran away to see a swan. It was hardly *that* much.

At least there is no sense of panic or concern these days, just a vague confusion, as though I've forgotten something. That's how it starts today as I sit at my desk. That's how the bad ones always start. I wander to the living room, frowning. Time has gone wrong. It is thick, catching on things, dragging its feet. I sit and stay still in its clumsy stumble, feeling the pressure of its hands. I realise I've been sitting here staring for, how long? An hour? Maybe time has got stuck in me and that is what I feel.

It takes work to remember you are safe. I try to do the work. There is a wood pigeon cooing in the gutter above the window. My son's black school shoes crisscross on the mat. I forget when I last polished them, but just thinking about that helps to ground me again. It takes an age to cross the room to lift the kettle, and I abandon it on its cradle, leaving it boiling as I crawl up to bed.

The world begins to tip, my vision to black and blur. I duck at the glare of the landing light, my eyes unable to adjust to light quickly, if at all. I begin to *feel* sounds, not hear them, like tuning forks held against me. The pigeon continues to call, each soft coo landing on my skin. A rumbling lorry approaches the corner outside awkwardly, navigating the parked cars. At some point soon, I know I will feel my bowel or my bladder cramp and loosen and have to go, go now. I begin to faint as I move, slumping until I am in a position where I can safely come and go like a tide, my head on the landing carpet, yesterday's washing on the ceiling airer high above me.

I feel it in my ears, my mouth, my head, the back of my neck. Fatigue comes in a wave and staying awake, keeping myself conscious, becomes painful. Somewhere under the weight of it, there comes an awareness that I've nodded off right there on the floor. I am glad my son isn't home.

I know to remain calm in the middle of all this now, stuck inside this body that has lost control. There is no panic and it's not so bad, not really. When days like this happen around him, I can still feel my usual, cheerful good nature through the fog of it, although making thoughts hold together becomes harder and my dumb jokes struggle to find their words. I try to hide it, as best as I can, but I forget how to do very simple things and must speak my intentions aloud step by step to guide me, speech thick, tongue clumsy. I feel stupid. Of course he notices. 'Why don't you have a lie down, Mummy?' he'll often say, and I hear him say it in memory now as I drift on the day. My bed is five feet away. I swim for the surface to make it there. There, I can let it pull me back under and doze while my body rages, loud and furious, my heart pounding in my chest.

I can do nothing but lie in shadow until the episode passes. Lying flat helps. Sometimes just doing that is enough to feel the sensation lift a little and I will laugh at the ceiling in relief at my body's absurdity, but it can often take the whole day to recover, two days, more. When my thoughts are clear enough, I meditate, counting breaths. Sometimes, but not often, I will have a good cry. Today, once I can, I will rise and take photos of the way the light catches the leaves of my houseplants, for the light is as still as I am today, and I feel grateful that I can make something good with it.

Every day feels different. Today brings with it a deep shame that this is my life and a biting sense of exclusion, the world hurrying by outside without me again. Often it is hard to believe I have anything of worth to say or to give, that I could ever be enough for anyone or anything, but the way to beat shame and the fear of rejection it hides is to make it all visible, to shake it all out somewhere spacious. Screw fear to hell.

Pay attention, be brave, see the truth, write it down. That will always be enough.

Tomorrow will be different again.

★

THEN

It wasn't all illness. There were long weeks in between of relishing in the pink light of my best friend Charlotte's bedroom, posters of ballerinas neat on her walls, where I would get to sleep on the floor some weekends and wonder, chest full, if she loved me as much as I loved her. Weeks of admiring her dozens of Barbie dolls and the pretty cascade of her hair. Weeks of pedalling up and down the pavement on my beloved red bike, of playing forgotten games with the rag-tag bunch of neighbourhood kids at 'the logs' at the bottom of our street.

The three sawn logs had been arranged at angles to make a balance beam on a scruffy, grassy, unbuilt-on space – a mockery of a playground, but it was our world just the same. My brother and I would be allowed to go there on our own and I'd walk there with my head high, racing ahead of him, stopping to hitch up the greying white of my long socks to glare at him impatiently, all of the previous week or month's pain forgotten. He'd trail behind me through the hours of each long day, as younger brothers do, asking over and over if I'd play with him. When the other kids were busy and I forgot my haughtiness, I'd say yes, and we'd have more fun together than I ever found with anyone else back then. I'd forget that the next day though, of course, and be back to rolling my eyes at him, wanting him to leave us older ones alone.

We'd all walk to school up and down past the same ex-council houses with their identical gates and small squares of mowed lawns. Summer playtimes on the big schoolfield seemed to fill whole afternoons as we made nests in the grass clippings or staged long marriage ceremonies between my complicated, dramatic classmates. The younger children would run and jump into my arms and wrap their thin legs around mine and I'd heave them around, delighted. 'You can be bridesmaid,' I'd say, grandly, and forget the business of marriage to make daisy-chain crowns until the bell was rung.

The sofa days would feel like a bad dream. The good grass stained my knees green, my worn checked dress, and any upsets were transient and fickle, soon spent. I wanted to be an actress, I declared. In church, I'd sing and sing.

'It's probably viral,' the doctor would say, the next time, frowning at my notes, 'but we should check her blood again.'

The tests would always come back normal, or close enough.

'Do you enjoy school?' they'd say, each time. 'How about friends? Have you anything on your mind?'

★

It has been a strange day of muttered portents and grumbled warnings. The first snow flurries fall more like ash than snow, settling in dry clumps and sticking to coats and eyelashes. Most folk are expecting a burying later this week and the same conversation is playing out everywhere I go, all eyes dark and pointed skywards.

'I heard that . . .', and, 'the forecast said . . .' I edge in and out of it on my scooter as I move about the small, familiar territory of my day. Community centre, corner shop, school playground; the same words delivered gravely from different, chapped faces, all buttoned up to their chins; the same barked dismissals from those determined to stand apart. 'What a fuss', and, 'it'll all come to nothing, just you mind,' back and forth.

The only thing anyone seems able to agree on is that it is damn cold and in that, in the end, there is at least some peace.

★

THEN

On the better days, I'd wander around our small garden trying to work out where it finished and I began. The garden was my mum's domain. I'd sit at the dining table by the window doing my homework and watch as the round shape of her benevolent, denimed behind bent over the flowerbeds, trowel in hand, but I'd wait until she'd gone inside to make our tea before I ventured out myself. I liked the hush of early evening the best. The motorway roared its soft roar. The long, thin poplar trees behind the back fence waved in the breeze.

I was ten now. I had watched the seasons change over and over, sitting in the same place at the same table. This was my home, and home was surely the same as me – I could hardly imagine us as separate things – but the garden had its own, murky edges and they weren't quite as safe as I felt they should be. They needed watching.

Certain places in the garden made me shiver, whatever the time of year. I would have to stand tall to build up the little inner push they required to be bolder, to go right to the edges of myself. Down the narrow side passage of the house in deep shade, thick with shrubs that offered dirty hollows to crawl into, if you didn't mind the dim, dry compression of it, or to the space under the old apple tree that smelled of rot and the stagnant water in the rain barrel. There was the gap too, between the dilapidated garage at the back and the fence, too small to squeeze through but visible enough to offer a long, forbidden corridor all the same. One to peer down, suspiciously because you couldn't quite see the end of it.

Other places offered easier sanctuary and I was reassured by them – reassured that some good things always stayed the same. The greenhouse smelled always of tomatoes. The concrete path wove always in the same display of curves and steps – I would check by walking it with my eyes closed. The compost heap always felt a little warm if you hovered your hands above it, and the names of the plants never changed, even when the winter tore them down. My mum taught me the names slowly, year by year, when I asked, 'what's this one? And this?' Hydrangea, fuchsia, forsythia, hosta, marigold, wallflower. I repeated their names to myself, silently, and said my own name alongside, trying to work out who I was and what on earth was happening to me.

★

I had asked my friend who lives by the sea to send me a pebble.

I will admit it: some days, I feel broken. Like a wave is broken. Not damaged, just scattered. The kind of lonely that makes you feel stretched so thin, you stop being able to see yourself.

I see very few people I know well week to week, month to month – almost no one, in fact beyond my son and Jude, and Mum and sometimes Dad – and although I value my solitude, it is hard. The people in my life do the best they can. I try not to demand too much because everyone else is stretched thin too, but I am learning to speak my simple needs in clear words when it matters and to remember that no one person can be everything I need. And so, I had asked a friend from Twitter for the pebble when they mentioned going for a walk along the beach. I saw a chance to hold something more real than I felt.

The envelope arrives today. In it, the smoothest, whitest stone. To press my thumb to it leaves a narrow halo of white. I put it in my pocket. It doesn't leave my side all day.

Talisman. I reach for it over and over. I reach for it as I watch the snow begin to fall in thick, ominous flakes outside; as I text the mum of my son's best friend, panicked, knowing my scooter wheels will get stuck in even half an inch; as I sit, miserable, on the stool in the kitchen dipping toast into my soup as the snow falls faster and faster, knowing I won't be able to leave the house now or see anyone else for days. I reach for it and soothe myself in the repetitive, uncomplicated way that children soothe themselves.

The pebble is a gift to sing over, as a medicine woman would. Sometimes my fingers find it icy; other times, it is inexplicably pulsing with warmth, even in the coldness of the day. I think it might have its own private moods, like I do, and I wonder if it is still joined to the tide that tumbled it somehow, reflecting that faraway edge. It is a link to a bigger life, to something wild.

I rub my thumb against it and try to picture the atoms of it, impossibly compressed into something still and enduring. My small new companion has been squeezed and heated beyond imagining, rising, sinking, re-forming, tumbled across millennia, all to end up a white star in my friend's gaze on the right day, in the right place when I needed it most, and if such things are possible, then anything is.

Holding it brings a sudden knowing. It doesn't matter if it's snowing. It doesn't matter if I can't get

out. I can sit here and the whole world can find its
way to me. Endless atoms and molecules, decaying,
circling, renewing: snow, water, stone, cloud, conifer,
bird. Who knows what they were all before, but
they're here now. I remember Rilke's poem from his
Book of Hours: 'How surely gravity's law, strong as an
ocean current, takes hold of the smallest thing and
pulls it toward the heart of the world . . .'

How simple it all feels now! There is no need
to be a tourist and I do not need to panic. I can
see every building block of this life if I sit right
here and wait for it to appear and know it when it
does. And I can do that. I am patient and watchful
enough. I am kind enough not to see anything as
unimportant. And wouldn't there be good company
in that? In me entertaining the whole of existence
come to visit?

Maybe if I sit still long enough, I can be an axis
around which every wonder spins.

Try thinking these thoughts and still feeling small
and alone and isolated, I dare you.

★

THEN

The metal frame of my hospital bed was covered
in stickers of gold stars. The nurses had begun the
custom of them to help me with my fear of needles.

I had to have blood tests every day, twice sometimes, and every time I got through one valiantly, a new star was fixed above my head. I was eleven and would have claimed to be too old for these things, but it worked all the same. I'd lie looking up at them, my bloody constellation, and knew that no one could tell me I wasn't brave now: I had proof. That bed was my home for only three weeks but, after the first, I felt like I'd been there forever.

The pain in my legs had grown so intense, I could barely walk. The usual doctor visit had turned, unexpectedly, into a referral to someone more senior. Scans showed my leg bones had thinned, considerably, inexplicably, although my muscles had not. Eyebrows were raised, letters sent. They cast the worst leg in plaster to stop it breaking and admitted me to the paediatric ward of our local hospital to control the pain while they puzzled over the unlikelihood of it all.

My heart hammered in my chest, but no one could see that. I had one job to do, and that was to be brave and earn my stars. No one needed to know that I was terrified, that my endless calm was a front, a mask. That would have only complicated the issue, and God knows, it was complicated enough.

★

Writing is about the only useful thing I know how to do from bed or a chair. I try to keep coming up with ways to make some use of it, to earn what money I can. Sometimes, my writing feels like hopeless desperation: a panic attack on paper. Other times, I am calm and convinced of some hidden direction, words sharp and confident. It barely keeps us afloat financially, but it allows me to avoid claiming long-term sickness benefits and to bypass their punishing restriction and judgement. It unlocks a world of learning for me to fall into. I write and I know I will learn how to write better. That gives me a life.

My latest money-making idea is essays in the form of letters. In them, I write about wonders: about extraordinary, overlooked things, to entertain and to nudge people into paying attention to what's around them. I post them directly to people who sign up for them online, people all over the world. They make a change from the constant stream of digital content. My letters are personal and secret and make people feel part of something. They have proved to be popular and once a month, I spend at least one full day hand-writing the envelopes.

Today would be a good day to make a start, I decide. My school-mum friend has promised to do all the school runs for as long as I'm stuck inside, however many snowy days we get, so I've got all day. I pull the lists of names and addresses and a box of envelopes into bed with me to work through while I keep warm. The world outside my window is white. It fills the room with hard, unusual light.

For hours, I rest a hand on the stack of papers filled with the names of people who have asked to receive my latest letter. I trace a finger down the line, touching each name and then letting the shape of it work up my arm and down the other. I doze and drift a little in between as I tire. I write each one with deliberate, cursive strokes, trying to let each name out in a single, smooth movement. I say the sound too, letting it fill my head as I make the marks, remembering that it holds a whole person inside of it. That's how you should write a name, I always think. That's the right way to do it. It is the names that make this task something to look forward to. I treasure every one.

Last night, I went to bed early with *A Wizard of Earthsea* by Ursula K. Le Guin who died last month and whose name and stories had bewitched me as a girl, lying in a different bed on the other side of town. It's been half a lifetime since I last read those books and yet every sentence, every image, feels familiar. Reading last night, I could remember the pull of excitement in my belly as I first read about Ged and the world of secret names he inhabited, names that could be known only through deep study or gifted in trust. I remember thinking, yes, this is what magic consists of, this true naming of a thing.

There is a turn in the tale when Ged first comes to the School of the Wizards and meets the Archmage of Roke, and the story goes like this:

In that moment Ged understood the singing of the bird, and the language of the water falling in the basin of the fountain, and the shape of the clouds, and the beginning and the end of the wind that stirred the leaves: it seemed to him that he himself was a word spoken by sunlight. Then the moment passed, and he and the world were as before, or almost as before.

It is a promise: a promise of what could be if he applies himself to his study of names and the nature of things. A glimpse of his potential and his future.

Whether it started with Earthsea, or with a dozen others, I can see now that I have spent much of my time since chasing what Ged felt in the courtyard at the beginning of his story. And the best of it all is that some days now, I *do* — I do feel like that, or close at least. There are moments when it feels like the thinnest of veils between me and everything else, that maybe with just the right kind of leap, I really could call down a sparrowhawk from the cold sky and call up each stone hidden under the snowdrifts by name. Words help me. That's why I write them.

It takes a long adult life to slowly shake off the magic you wish for and to discover the magic there is but gradually, you realise that it's all the same in either case.

Magic is simply seeing clearly and once you know that, even the mundane life you have been dealt – one of grotty side-streets, not enchanted islands – can feel like a scholarship at the school that you've always dreamed of. Then, the language of water, wind and dirty snow is just a matter of sitting and watching with a notebook and a pen, same as it was for all the wizards that came before you.

It all starts and ends with names, with words, taking the time to know things for what they are, and to appreciate them for that too.

These are the things I think as I write the names today, and each one feels like a word spoken by the sharp winter sun.

★

THEN

I'd lie in my star bed in a bay with five other children and watch people come and go. I remember a younger girl who spent long hours on a nebuliser, the dry hiss wandering over to dry my mouth too when she fidgeted and it slipped; a toddler whose nose always ran green and who had his legs fixed and splayed in full leg casts, blue and angry.

The hospital was like a giant fish tank. I'd hear the sounds as though underwater, tired or drugged or bored. Hushed, focused voices; only occasionally the sharp jolt of a laugh. The adults talked one at a time, out of sight at the desk around the corner, and I'd strain to try and recognise the voices of nurses I loved best, hoping they were on shift. I still remember some of their names: Pat, Sarah, Julie.

Phone pulse. Trolley rattle. The porters you'd know instantly because they spoke twice as loudly as everyone else and whistled their way through the ward. I floated in my tank and the dry, solid world outside on the other side of the glass looked hard and strange. We drew faces on paper plates and stuck them on the window. We made them with Siân the play therapist, colouring them sad, scared or cheerful to show how we were feeling, or thought we should. I remember those plates, that the light through the window made them glow.

I remember I cried with homesickness, quietly, in the sickly pulse of the night lights. I didn't want to wake the others. I didn't want to make a fuss. I missed my little brother. I missed our garden. I missed my white bedroom: a warmer, safer white than this one.

★

It is a strange week. The snow persists and makes a canvas of everything and I sit and watch it. As more of the land is buried, the opposite seems to happen to people. Everyone seems to melt back to something habitual, everyone becoming a caricature of themselves.

I can't help but turn to social media when I'm feeling particularly stuck. I abandon my work and reach for my phone and watch the country react to what's happening outside, scrolling down through each expression. In Twitter missives, in posted photos, I see us all pared back to some secret core. All of life's well-worn attitudes come in a digital avalanche.

I see people online dismiss the snow, determined to make it small and trivial. Others seem bent on stressing its bigness, its competitive covering, as if to have the most in their area is to have won. I see those who speak only of the joy of it, who are made children by it, and those who can feel only its hardships.

Through the window of my phone, I see bravado and daring, boasts of conquests and defiance against weather's so-called warnings. I see softer, humbler, endurance. Shouted, ego-plumped demonstrations of charity towards older people and the homeless run alongside quieter, overlooked kindnesses, while others sit back and argue about which is more important.

I see those using the snow as just another backdrop to stress the sensuality of their bodies. I scroll past photos of long, bared legs carefully posed against the snowy backdrop (the mother in me tutting and worrying for their health) to see blurry snaps of those who have embraced only the ridiculousness of themselves and the circumstance, wearing silly hats to sledge their way down hills on bin bags. I see people become artists as they take and share considered photographs of laden trees, of transformed landscapes. Meticulously sculpted igloos take their place alongside cock-and-balls scrawls drawn large on car windows.

I see people take on the role of snow's spokespeople, telling us what we should do about it, and notice those who hardly mention it at all. Some post long essays debating what this extreme cold spell means, for our futures, for our climate, while others seem concerned only about themselves, only looking out to the world in order to retreat to the easy comfort of consumerism, panic buying supplies from the supermarket.

Some emphasise restriction and restlessness while others seem free, but each of us reacts to some need, all framed by the snow. Same event: a hundred different stories.

As for me, I overthink it all more than is necessary, of course, for I am as predictable as the rest. I worry about the small, frail bodies of birds and the limbs of trees, and the bodies and limbs of people too, until at last the snow stops, and begins to melt.

I had imagined the thaw would come like something fresh and certain. Instead, it comes as dishwater: grey and full of last week's slops. I breathe a sigh that holds relief and confusion all in one because I have hated the added restriction of the last week, unable to get out even to the community centre, but have loved having something new to look at.

Now it's disappearing, most people have moved on to other things already. But stuck where I am, the slush still too thick for my scooter wheels, my fingers still scrolling for company, for connection, I find I can see the same reactions and instincts online, the same deep expressions of self played out over and over, muddy in the meltwater. There was nothing new in any of it, not really. We simply all used the same canvas for a little while: the white made an easy one.

I keep thinking that there is something beautiful and fragile and desperate about the whole thing. How predictable we become when we lose some control. How very fleeting all this is.

★

THEN

A long stream of consultants visited, their minions with notebooks like reporters at a press conference.

They discussed the data of me coolly, unimpressed. I remember the name of only one, who sat on the bed and held my hand as he addressed his congregation to remind me that whatever the words sounded like, he still saw me there, smiling, terrified. He was the orthopaedic surgeon and his name was Mr Gwynn, and I loved him because he held my hand and because his name sounded like a word from an Arthurian legend. The rheumatologist was wide and bosomy and spoke with an accent I hadn't heard before, and I didn't like her at all because it was she who seemed to want all my blood, endlessly, and who never seemed to be satisfied with what she saw there. The urologist's student passed me cardboard bowls I was supposed to fill, and I'd pass them back through the toilet door balanced on one leg, braced and blushing, my yellow offerings softening them and marking a dark line around the rim.

I was tired, and my legs hurt like they always did, but when misery burned away with the morning, I ended up enjoying the bustle of hospital life. There were so many people to watch: it was miles better than a sofa. Suddenly, I had more visitors than I'd ever had before. After a while, friends from school came, my teachers too sometimes, even though it was the summer holidays. I felt reassured that I hadn't broken anything with my absence after all.

I learnt to cross stitch – I think someone must have brought me a kit – and spent the time littering the white sheets with a rainbow of snipped threads. One of the nurses smuggled me some disposable surgical scissors, wrapped in plastic, to cut them with. They were blue handled, precise and perfect: a treasure I kept for years after.

I had my first period in that star bed, unprepared and unexpected, early for my age, staining the white, starched sheets with a neat circle of red. Hardly anything; barely a flower. I wore the thick hospital pad between my legs, my face even redder than its hidden secret, and wondered if this was what life was like for everyone, to live in a body that had its own mind, that was obviously not mine, because it couldn't be, could it?

I had not decided on any of this, I promise, I wanted to say, to my parents, to my friends, to the doctors. You have to believe me. I didn't mean for any of this to happen.

★

Long hours are spent propped up in my bed as this winter finally runs itself out. From here, I can see through the window to the grubby backstreet that leads to the sheltered housing complex and then to the community centre. My view is of stiff, red-bricked chimneys and drunk garden fences, bleached by weather. The grey house opposite makes a thick stripe down the right-side edge of my window and the space to its left frames the one lone tree that has worked its way through the hard scrub of the pavement's edge. My lime tree. Soon, I will watch it swell and turn green, blocking the sky, but for now, for only a little while longer, it is still all finger and bone.

A shape appeared in its branches last week, sagging red and limp from a lower limb. For days, I have guessed it to be debris from the bad weather, or something careless and putrid, knotted and tossed there by someone who doesn't give two shits but had collected one. It is only today that I manage to get over to see what it is.

It's a bird feeder. I find four of them. Cheap and cheerful Poundshop fare: a coconut filled with fat strung up in the hoary underbrush, and others like the red seed-feeder I had spied zip-tied and dotted around the lower branches.

Riotous charms of goldfinches and long-tailed tits career their way around these streets, blue tits and great tits too. I hear each individual song from my bed. I have learnt them, so I would know them. Sparrows in the gutters and wrens in the hedges, chaffinches and greenfinches in the untidy conifers, all small and as chaotic as the rest of us.

Someone here, nearby, must know them as I do, know that they will be hungry, know that they will be nesting very soon. Someone without a garden, for they are a rare commodity here, must have also sat and worried about frail bodies and hungry beaks during the snow. They must have made their way out in the snow and bought the feeders and hung them like baubles over the dirty pavement. Bright offerings to life and care and remembering.

Whoever you are, I love you.

I will never stop being surprised by how *good* life is. I will never stop being surprised at the tenderness we hide.

★

THEN

'The good news is, she doesn't have bone cancer,' one of the white coats said one day, and everybody who loved me cried. I hadn't even realised that was what they were looking for. I wasn't even entirely sure what cancer was, but I knew it was bad, so I was glad, glad I didn't have this bad name that even the absence of made my mother weep.

In the end, they simply booked a date for me to have the sensory nerves to my lower legs blocked, to help numb some of the pain. Now I could focus on getting back on my feet, they said, back on track to start high school in the autumn. I'd stay in hospital only a little while longer: this wasn't the place for me now, they agreed. Nobody said why it had happened. Nobody seemed to know. I guess that was the bad news.

So, I counted the days. I watched the ward. The little boy with his legs in traction wore white nappies and greying vests, and his face was always red and puffy from crying. He'd whine and whine and some nights, I would hate him. Other times, the odd time there was a wheelchair left next to my bed after a trip to the toilet, I would swing my legs out of bed and wheel myself over to him to pull faces and make him smile. I didn't know what you were supposed to do with three-year-olds, what you were supposed to say, and so I'd just make my face like rubber, puffing out my cheeks and screwing up my eyes until he laughed.

They'd never let me keep the wheelchair for long now, in case I 'got used to it'. I remember those words. I'd look at it, worried, wondering how it might trap me. I did like sitting in it, it was true, and racing along the long corridors like a carrier pigeon for a change. I felt guilty for that.

Instead, the physio walked me up and down the corridor next to my bed, once a day. I'd inch my way along the floor, balanced on my crutches, every step a little explosion. They'd nod and smile – good, good girl – and I'd puff up with confused pride. I remember crying long, silent tears that leaked out of me in streams. I'd wipe them away as soon as they sprung, pausing in my progress to rub at them fiercely. I so wanted to be good. I would sleep and sleep afterwards, waking, feverish, with the soft press of a thermometer to my ear ('just doing your obs, pet'), to the rattle of the dinner trolley, the gradual arrival of visitors to other beds marking the open hours, until, one day, finally, I was deemed well enough to leave.

Everything looked wrong when I got home. I would touch things, wonderingly, trying to remember when they used to feel familiar. The crutches rubbed under my armpits and the rubber handles made my nose wrinkle, but I did my best to get the rhythm of them. The uncast leg hurt a little less, and so I'd lean on that one, and scoot the other forward. And once the nerve blocks were done, it did get a little easier, although I didn't walk well again without crutches or a curved walking stick for at least another year after that and even then, there were always the unexpected, inexplicable bad days that would make me limp and lurch.

'Hopalong Cassidy' people would call me. I hadn't got a clue what it meant but would smile anyway because they seemed to mean it nicely.

★

The slush has finally eased enough to get out to the community centre again. I catch sight of myself in the car windows as I pass. There is no getting around it: I do not look good this winter. I am pale and drawn, slightly jaundiced, like something you'd find somewhere damp and dark. My eyes are swollen, shrunken small, eye bags bruised and heavy, my short hair brittle and rapidly flecking grey. I've been particularly unwell for months now; one infection after another. I exist, misshapen, made bloated by thick jumpers and my winter coat, hunched by fatigue. To come face to face with people in the street is to have them pull back a little, through surprise and concern. I am no one's fantasy just now and would laugh loud at any attempt to make me so.

There is an unexpected freedom in it, in shaking off prettiness for a while, like something extra and unnecessary. I simply have no energy left to pretend or preen. I do not look good because my body is sick and why should it be expected to make beauty when it is tired and fighting hard? I don't owe anyone a pretty face. That is not my required payment to the world, nor to anyone to prove my worth, and knowing this makes me love my friendly bones harder. I scoop myself up like a mangy old cat, all scars and patchwork, wanting to bring warmth and care to those ugly parts that life tells me I should be horrified by.

I am beginning to understand those old, bent women who dance, who shake the wrinkled sheets of their spotted arms, who let their low breasts sway.

I am beginning to see the exhausted, obstinate sense in it. Why be pretty when you can be everything else?

There is something pure and perfect about ugliness. There is something mutinous in it. It comes free of sentimentality and delusion and all the other things we crowd around beauty, adoringly, until we can barely see it at all. Ugliness is plain and stark and true and joyful, when you let it be. And I feel it, worn out as I am. I feel the simplicity and wholeness of being uncovered like this because there is still so much room for love.

Love is not excluded when beauty leaves. If anything, it finds a new kind of power. Yes, to come face to face with people is to have them pull back a little at first, but I have noticed that those who love me most then move a little closer in response. My son does, even Tina in the community centre kitchen does. What tenderness there is in that. What happy connection. I know that good things can still grow here.

It makes me look at ugly things again, at the rich compost of last year's brown leaf mulch in the gutters and the slumped mess of snow's weight on the verges. I smile with a secret knowing. There is power in decay and I claim it.

Besides, I can be ugly and still write like a dream. What on earth does it matter?

★

THEN

The priest from our church came to visit me sometimes. In the hospital, at home. There must have been more than one priest, now that I think about it, but it always went the same way and so they blur together. I'd sit, obliging as always, and screw up my eyes tight as he put a calloused hand on my hair and said fierce words of denouncement, of banishment. I felt like he was ordering God, not asking him, and I was awed at his confidence.

After the stronger statements, he'd slip into the strange, lyrical rush of sounds that I knew was called speaking in tongues. That meant the Holy Spirit had got inside him. They'd say it was like feeling a summer wind blow through you when it happened. It always sounded beautiful to me and I wished I could do it too, jealous of the teenagers at church who could, while the adults looked on proudly. I never could, though, my tongue forever an obstinate plank in my mouth. I'd sit and try and make the sounds, the belief hot in my chest, my fists clenched tight against my thighs with the effort, and I'd try and try, but I never felt anything, not really.

I'd pray, though, often, eyes closed, wondering if someone was listening; terrified that maybe they were but had simply turned away. By the time I was eleven, my dad had lost his faith. The depression had receded like a tide and, slowly, he had realised that faith was not left on the cluttered beach of him. My mum still tried, to pray, to believe. She gave it everything. Everyone we knew wanted a miracle for the pale, limping child in their congregation – I was ripe for one – but I, awkward, unchosen, failed to deliver. The shame of that was deep and enduring.

Years later, in runs of better months when I walked better, looked bright, I'd bump into grey-haired, soft-eyed old ladies, who had once handed out hymnbooks and arranged harvest festival tins, and their delight to see me dripped with triumph. How happy they were that God had finally got around to me after all!

I'd ignore the age-old ache in my legs as they told me how well I looked. You don't like to be a killjoy, do you?

★

My camera, oh, my magic third eye. It is my comfort blanket. Other days, a shield, a wall. On days when I feel too visible or too unwell, it lets me put something between the obviousness of my difficulty and everything else, but with it in my hands, I can still reach out and touch things; everything.

Some days, I feel more tree than person: a wilder god than the one I was taught about, one long since forgotten. I can't join in much, but I'm learning to ride the energy of others better and let it carry me to those places and experiences I can't reach. I listen and watch and try and take it all in as my own.

Every day, I am learning how to be apart and still belong. It is not an easy thing, especially with my son still young, still full of play. The trick is to carry the grief lightly. It is hard not to mourn the don't-see and don't-do and instead celebrate the victory of second-hand experience, but you can do it, if you can just put bitterness to one side and love what you receive instead. My boy helps. He is living a good life. He is happy. Today we wrap up warm and Mum takes us to the park. Leaving me safe in my wheelchair, they run off to enjoy the day, throwing a frisbee against the cold wind.

It is in this place, here at the edge, that my camera finds its meaning. It lets me push my eyes up close, to watch faces, gestures, movement, and bring something back, even though I am separate. And there is so much to be found here. Not from intrusively tunnelling somewhere I don't belong, but from joining it considerately, part of a conversation.

I focus in and in and change my size, shrinking until I can walk down the cracks in the path and peer up at walls towering a hundred feet above me. I stretch myself until I can swallow the whole sky, the daytime moon, every tree in sight, greedily seeing how much I can hold. I leap with another slide of the zoom, taking myself wherever I wish, perching on rooftops and branches, following birds right into their new nests.

With my camera in my hands, I am omnipotent, free, and there are no barriers between me and the making of something good and true and permanent. Pain can't interrupt it, and neither can my dwindling mobility because there is nearly always something right where I am. I only need to sit and look and raise the lens, just like I only need to keep my hand moving across a blank page to write. Everything that matters can come from those two things and neither can be taken away from me. My health can't steal words or pictures, and neither can poverty or heartbreak or anything else. There is triumph in that.

And when my physicality does get too much, with photographs I can simply disappear entirely, hiding myself like a code in the arrangement of a picture and its secret heart. I can make all my energy visible in that; no one needs to know I remain slumped and tired. I can share my pictures rather than myself.

When speech won't come now, it doesn't matter. I can close my mouth and instead let myself be this caressing, loving eye that sees perfection and beauty in everything, in every place. I can take photos and turn the camera back around to the world, to my son and my mother, and say look, look how perfect you are.

★

THEN

High school was not easy on crutches. I started there late, a few weeks after my hospital admission, not yet twelve. I was a diminutive first year, under-formed, unevolved, and the school was big, rough and wild – notorious, even, in our small, uninteresting West Midlands town. It had given me a thrill of excitement to learn that, before I went, as if it somehow might make me wilder by association, but it was the only secondary school in our neighbourhood so that was that. I readied myself to be changed, inevitably, and wondered what it would feel like. Gentle, soft me waited to be made hard at last.

In the end, to be there was simply to be jostled, bored, unchallenged. There was a lethargy to its corridors, its weary teachers, the dirty cream of its walls. It didn't feel remotely special and I felt no different. I did what all first years did and tried to make myself as small as possible, flinching in my inability to do so, always taking up too much space. A dangerous amount of space, I took up, anomaly that I was.

Nobody seemed to have planned for a child who couldn't walk. An option wasn't provided to resent or question that, and, in any case, it didn't matter – it wasn't like I was disabled, I remember thinking, picturing plucky, smiling kids paralysed in special wheelchairs. It wasn't like this counted, and I assumed everyone else thought the same.

The classrooms stretched up and up in blocks three, four stories high, subjects housed in buildings spread wide from each other: a chaotic, concrete city. There were no ramps and the stairs were the hard, sharp kind that bruised your shins. Children cascaded down them like meltwater, like rocks, like wildebeests driven mad with fear, and my careful physio-trained, crab-like progress up and down them meant nothing to their huge, unseeing, unstoppable force.

I would stand frozen in the rush of it, gripping the handrail with both hands, clinging until the danger had passed and then continue, shaking, in pain. Was I meant to be going up or down? Making my way to a lesson late, or retreating from one early?

I don't remember many lessons. I existed on the stairs. They were red, red like a tongue, like something slipped and broken. I am not ashamed to tell you how afraid I was. Me, with my brave face and my endless will. I was not easily cowed, but this was a real and necessary terror. When I picture them, the stairs shine like something wet, glistening with just melted slush, or from a just-passed wave. I wanted rope, guide, tether. Anything. Anything.

I would often collapse halfway and have to sit on them, trying to pull myself into the sides and the corners, defeated, while muffled lessons continued around me, above me.

★

The cold rain wakes my son and me. It sounds angry. I am angry too. I had fallen asleep excited by the next day's work. I had so many ideas; so many things to say, but now, today, I can do nothing but feel ill and what use is that to anyone.

We huddle under the umbrella on our way to school, me trying to steer the scooter with one hand and hold the umbrella with the other, my son keeping pace at my side. Hunched and grumpy, we resent the darkness and the rain with every angle of our backs that we can stiffen. The primary school playground always floods and so we wait in the lake that has formed. From under my hood, all I can see are legs: grey flamingos, all of us tucking in as much of ourselves as we can manage.

Back home, my spinal cord is something molten, my hands ice, and I press one to the back of my neck, grateful. It eases the hot pulse. My arms are carrying the strange, numb vibration of the faint that came when I woke up. I feel full of something. I grasp for metaphors: a swarm of dark bees, shadowy thunder clouds, something shifting, pulsing. I know I will get nothing done today.

Reason tells you that pain is something held entirely inside yourself, but after a while, you know better. There are weeks when intense pain, the kind you've

long carried, leaks out to coat everything around you.
Some balance tips and the container of you overflows.
It grows bigger than you are, and you cannot hold it
in and so it starts to ooze out. I am often amazed to
pull myself up and see I haven't left my chair dripping
with the tar of it. Even the air around me has felt thick
and visceral lately, like I must be filling that too. To
move, to think, is to have to push into it and through
it. It is so tiring. I am so tired.

Self-pity is the opposite of outward attention. You
turn your mind inwards and close all the doors to the
outside as you go, carefully pushing out everything that
doesn't relate directly to your pain, until all that's left is
this one dark tunnel to peer down, nothing but your
own suffering at the bottom. Of course you can't help
but look. You've forgotten there is anything else to do.

It is an inevitable habit, understandable and human.
I can't avoid it, not entirely, but I am at least beginning
to embrace the reverse more often now: the long
breath followed by the faint whirr as the trap is
released, as something else turns you by the shoulders,
as the doors open around you. It's in these moments
that the world is remade.

It is Jonas that does it today. Because I spend my
life lower to the ground than other adults, children
talk to me; little brothers, little sisters. Back in the
playground for pick-up time, he bobs up next to my
scooter missing both top front teeth and delights in

demonstrating that he can no longer say his own name, all esses lost to him for the foreseeable (or the foretheeable, if you are Jonas). The wind hisses around him as he laughs and tries over and over, as if it is whipping the sound right out of his mouth, and with that, all is changed.

The name lost, I look at the grinning boy still in front of me, whole and wonderful. I remember that pain isn't poison, however it feels. It is deep and sharp, but it can move through you and do no harm. It is something other than me, other than all of us. I can hold it like black air, like noise or wind or a wild sea or the weather, but it isn't my shape. It isn't what I'm made of. It means nothing more than a storm or a single, shifting night.

I am not the weather. I am the wide and open sky, and so I can let pain move through me and out of me. The air isn't thick with oil or smog or something bad pouring from me; it is simply the wind of a dark day that I can lean into until it passes. 'Pain, you can't hurt me,' I whisper as Jonas dashes off, and I laugh because the words are absurd and because they're true.

★

THEN

A decision was made that I was a danger to everyone, or perhaps that I was the one in danger – I don't remember which it was. I was put in the corner of the Home-Ec room, where I hungrily watched an endless procession of sagging Victoria sponge cakes and shepherds' pies make their awkward way into being. Work was brought to me sometimes but not always. The Home-Ec teacher was white-haired and red-faced, as all women of her role are, and she made a noise like a bag being sat on when she looked at me, although she would, sometimes, in her better moods, offer me plates of leftover biscuits in the lull between her noisy, resistant classes, and I liked her then.

I was bored. Bored beyond imagining. I had never been as bored before or since. I might well be the one of the cleverest girls in my primary school, they had once delighted in telling my parents that loudly over the top of my head, despite all my time off – I would go far, I had POTENTIAL, they had said – but now I sat on an unsteady stool by a cooker using a textbook to try and teach myself algebra. I didn't feel angry then, just sad and afraid. I had never felt comfortable with all that praise anyway, always feeling like it was a mistake somehow, and now, look, I was right. I had let everybody down. I tried hard not to think about it, but it was like a mosquito in the room.

I left for lunch early, returned early, listening to the stampede I had avoided with a mixture of relief and grief. The friends I'd made soon found others to fill the space I'd taken. Friendships then were fickle to form and easy to break and loyalty could turn with the day, let alone with a month, three, six.

The whole first year passed in a blur.

★

I take the long way home today. I take my time.

The thing is, if you can leave loneliness at the door, there are days when solitude can feel like a bright dream. It takes on a sort of thrum: something full, reverberant. It helps to let go of resentment first, especially the secret, hoarded kind. I'm getting better at that, slowly. It helps more if I can stop thinking I'm owed something. Then the world can pour in to fill the space I've left for it.

I don't think madness would feel this quiet. I don't think mysticism would feel this ordinary. I have learnt to slip between the two, unnoticed and undemanding.

It's a good place to find, if you can. Here, for a while at least, you get to be nothing but you, watching the crows in the trees. You get to be that simple and that extraordinary.

★

THEN

One day, late in that first year, just before the summer holidays, a boy I had cradled a crush on for long years said 'stop right there a minute' to me as I made my slow way along the corridor to the dining hall, and I did, obediently, confused, balancing on my crutches as best I could.

He pulled a girl I didn't know towards him – round-faced, fair and pretty – and he kissed her, loudly, wetly, unpractised, a foot from my face. I blushed scarlet as the crowd around them laughed and ran off, not understanding the point they were making but also understanding utterly, deep down. Unkissed. Unchosen. Newly awake with something, something.

I felt it somewhere new, too. Somewhere deep and pulling. A clock was ticking.

★

I wish them both the happiest weekend. I say, 'Please send photos!' I pull my son close and tell him that I know he'll make the best ring-bearer in the world. And then I shut the door.

Today, my ex-husband will marry again and I will not. I wish him nothing but joy. That is a good thing to hold to your heart and know to be true.

My own unmarriedness feels correspondingly bigger for the change. I find myself newly self-conscious of my solitary nature. I had not given it much thought in recent years until suddenly, these last few weeks, the wedding date looming, I did again. It is unusual to be on your own at thirty-six and not be looking for a somebody, I know that, and yet it's true and I am not. Dating culture left me cold and is not a game I want to play again. Besides, how on earth would I manage it now?

Love has found me more than once in the years since my marriage. Each time it was not in a shape I could keep or mould to my wanting despite my every effort to squeeze it until it was. I have tried to love in return, fiercely, tenderly, but whether through fate or habit, it has never found its mark in a soul who was able to give it a full home. There was always an *if*, always a *but*. Always something held back, in them, and in me sometimes, too: a distance or a mismatch or a line that couldn't be crossed. Always a gap.

I have grieved hard for that, at times, until I saw that what I grieved wasn't just what was lost but what I imagined *should have been*. In my sorrow, I had felt sure I'd been denied a wholeness. It took time to see the illusion of that. It took time to see it was a lie.

After a lifetime of determined, wilful jigsawing of lives, one day I stopped. I didn't want to do it any more. I stopped insisting to myself that I held a gap to be filled and that I should do everything I could to shore it up. I stopped believing, too, that the people I met were supposed to fit me.

The idea of some missing piece in me assumed that either the love I had found and lost was the wrong shape, or I was. A tempting dark hole of thought to

fall down at times, but although I know I am difficult
sometimes, I know I am not difficult to love. And what
an arrogance to think that the people I adored and the
things they offered were wrong somehow, just because
we couldn't come and stay together smoothly! No,
each was as it was, and all was right in its own way.
The best they could give was given, and the rest was
just how it was. The measure of something's goodness
isn't determined by how well it goes my way.

So, there is no searching out or sizing up of potential
mates these days, I just can't bear it. But where I once
imagined an absence that needed new love to fill it,
I now rejoice in finding older loves already there.
I have my friendship with Jude that is as enduring as
any marriage, while my deep passion for my work and
interests leaves me as distracted and obsessed as any
crush. And there is motherhood, of course: entirely
its own adventure in love. I relish my own time and
autonomy. What's more, in not looking, not hunting,
there is a peace that feels like sitting at home with the
doors wide open. There is more air here than I have
ever known. Things happen here.

I am neither so naive nor so jaded to think that love
won't find me again or that it can't ever last. I expect it
will, it's just that next time, I think it will feel differently.
When I picture it, I imagine absentmindedly throwing
something over my shoulder and turning to find
someone has caught it; us both smiling and saying

'oh.' I think it will feel like that – not a filling up, but an offering *out*. But, however it comes, I am not in any rush for it and I think that, more than anything, is what makes my solitude feel newly awkward.

I think, deep down, I am a little embarrassed at how much I am enjoying my life, especially when the world insists on telling me that I really shouldn't. And so today, here's to that: to my contented unmarriedness.

I look around my quiet, empty house, full of signs of myself and my boy and our life. Our photos on the wall, our daft, grinning selfies, my possessively full bookshelves, my sprawling knitting on the chair. No one else to decode, no one to negotiate with or try to impress, and I smile and smile and smile.

★

THEN

I don't remember when I first realised that the doctors thought I was mad or over-exaggerating or both. It seeped into me like cold damp: one of those things you don't notice until the day you happen to put a hand to it and your heart sinks. Whatever, whenever, the day came when I realised that's what they believed, and I thought my parents must believe it too. I thought everyone believed it. It felt like being found out and yet I was sure I hadn't done anything bad. Had I?

'We can't find anything really wrong with you.' Back at the GP's surgery after months more fatigue and pain, the words that would haunt me my whole life began to form a holy law. I began to bend myself to them, to become their pragmatic certainty. To be good. To be forgiven.

The words 'chronic fatigue' had been passed back and forth for years by then but it didn't seem to mean anything to anyone. They were just words to stop you asking again. 'It's her age. She'll grow out of it,' they said now I'd hit puberty, and I wondered why this age mattered when the others didn't. These days, I suspect the same thing will happen when I hit the menopause: it's always your age when you're a woman. In any case, everyone was tired. Tired of me saying I was tired. Perhaps the chronic fatigue was theirs – a description of what I had induced. Oh, but they were doing their best, I know that.

I knew I wasn't mad. At least, I didn't think I was. I knew about the dangerous kind of sadness and I had looked and looked since it had taken my dad away that time, but I couldn't seem to find it in me.

When I did feel sad or worried, I would freeze, wondering if this was it – had it found me at last? Worse: had it been in me all along? Maybe now was the moment it would start to spread, racing down the pathways the pain had made for it until it ate me from the inside out. Maybe that had always been its pathology. That's why the doctors always asked me how I was feeling about my life: they knew. They knew that's how it began to get you.

But, then, something would make me laugh. Even at my most overcast, I would laugh. That has never changed. Something would make me tip back my head and open my arms, my heart. Something else would be too interesting to keep me thinking about all this, about pain, about school, about boys who didn't like me. There would come a book, a project, a hobby, a thing I'd like to try. There was always something else to pull me away. There was an easy, curious joy in me always, undeterred, nudged right up against any sorrow and never diminished by it, although I rarely let anyone see that either. I was a tender, hidden thing, in pain and in love, for all of it, in everything.

★

A long time ago, I decided on the best day of the year in advance. I've found it takes the pressure off all the other days, knowing you've already got a best day picked out. Every other day can unravel however it needs, with no expectation for it to be anything special. Of course, it *can* be special if it wants to be, but you don't have to worry about it if it's not. You can remember last year's best day clearly and without conflict, look forward to the next, and all other days can fall contentedly behind.

The best day of the year is the day I hear the first blackbird of the year sing its low, sweet song. It is made all the better by the fact that you never know exactly when it will happen. You just have to wait and hope, but once you do, you know that spring is coming. Not yet, but soon.

Today is the day I hear it. It takes me and carries me and, for a moment, I know bliss.

The unexpected, sudden sunshine of the day must have filled his small, dark body up to the beak until he couldn't help but pour it out of him. And this during the briefest of moments when I just happen to be somewhere quiet and alone, my camera in my pocket, with a clear view of him and an undistracted eye. All aligned.

Three minutes later, he is gone, but it is enough, enough to catch a photo of him, yellow beak wide against blue sky, and mark my best day loud and clear. It doesn't matter what else the day held before it, or the week, or any other day carried heavily and for longer than was needed. It is a magic spell to wipe all clean, a hard reset, and I embrace it willingly with my heart wide open.

The blackbird sang and I let myself be as happy as I know how, without thought or complication, knowing this is my perfect day.

My year begins again then. I close my eyes. I cannot shake the smile of it.

If there is any kind of prayer left in me, I think this might be it.

★

THEN

On the days of too much, days when I could barely stand, could do nothing but lie trapped in my lead suit again, my legs compressed and burning with pain, the sand running out of me, I would try telling myself, firmly and determinedly: 'There is nothing really wrong with you.' The tests said so, the doctors said so, and I believed in truth, in the right thing. I didn't want to be a liar. Confusion and shame pulsed in me, a panicked white noise, but there was a certain righteous, relieved victory in choosing to believe them in the end, because doctors were right and good, I was sure of it.

I began to try and push through it more and more. I learnt to grit my teeth and close my fists and smile harder. I'd remember the physio in the hospital – how I was rewarded for my stoicism. I started to mention it all less and less, obliging in the advice to 'not feed the pain', worried too that, otherwise, it would spoil my goodness, my value.

I knew I was supposed to start becoming something new now anyway and I was desperate for that something to be accepted, desired, by the other girls at school, by my parents, by the older boy from our church that I had started to like in that deep, pulling way. He'd look at me sometimes, knowing, alien, and I'd feel my stomach expand and contract like a fish on the ground. I didn't know what they all wanted, but I knew it wasn't this.

I think I hoped that I could leave it all behind, all I'd been so far, along with Father Christmas and the ponies on the windowsill, the balancing logs down the road, the flower fairies I had once been sure lived under the forsythia.

I battled to reject the sensations of my body along with all those other things I wasn't supposed to need any more. Not wanting to act out, all I could do was swallow the lot and try and hold it still in my belly. It's only now I can see what else was displaced by its mass.

No. I mustn't look at it. It was like a bad child in class. I mustn't let it know I see it. Only then would it stop.

★

My son is properly unwell for the first time in ages, the end of the winter marking itself in him in one last, loud viral display. Alongside the instinctive clench of worry that comes when your children burn hot and pale and fold in on themselves like limp playing cards,

I try to remember that here is a chance to teach him things that will last his whole life.

You must learn how to be sick well. I want him to learn that getting sick isn't a punishment and that he won't be punished for being so. I usher in good rest and comforts instead. We laugh. We talk about what makes us feel better. How good it is that we can help each other to do these things! I want him to learn that he is not harder to love when he is inconvenient and so today I use all the words I know to show him that it's fine, this is not a bad time: we just need to do different things for a while. It probably won't be for long and how lucky is that?

I also want him to learn that life doesn't stop when illness moves in. I allow room for boring humdrum. My work and my needs continue and he has had to come up with his own entertainment and continue to help out and, yes, you absolutely still have to brush your teeth and do your homework, kiddo, even if you do them more slowly.

We sit together quietly, the TV a soothing burble of sound. When we feel like talking, we talk about what we need to do to take care of ourselves, about what happens in our bodies when we get sick because, god, that's amazing, isn't it? We talk about what we can do to help them, about what he can do and I can do – what we need from each other – and how it all goes best when we get the balance of that right. We talk about what it feels like to be unwell, *where* we feel it, and try to find the best descriptions to match up to our bodies, but we also talk about lots of other things because to talk about illness all the time gets boring.

Mostly though, we let our soft bodies rest against each other as often as we can, remembering that we are animals and need nests, food, sleep and each other. We fill our days with stories, because they are often the best and most reliable human medicine. Sick days should always be full of them, especially those with wizards in.

I tuck him into bed early tonight and his face is sad on the pillow. 'I'm so sorry it's been a hard day, Mummy,' he says, and I say I am sorry too because some days that's true and it's important to be honest about these things.

He falls asleep, leaving all the other redemptive words I want to say unspoken.

★

THEN

I began to lose something then. I dimmed and it was noticed. I began my second year at high school pale and silent and within a few weeks, my parents decided enough was enough. I was moved to a better school across town, where I could be stretched and where, they said, I would get the chance to be around kids who were more like me.

The uniform's ties featured woven white birds and the other kids would pull out the threads till they turned black. To my relief I now sat in the library rather than the Home-Ec room, with the new school still towering up impossibly high above me.

I stayed out of the way. I read my books. I filled in slightly harder worksheets. I waited, ever hopeful, hungry, vulnerable, every new breath of me swallowed back down, until one day, the boy from my church asked if I'd like to go to the cinema with him. And I said yes.

★

It's Thursday and we have come to Jude's for tea. I think about gentleness as I lie on her sofa and we talk about kindness. I think about it again as I scoot the three streets home in the dark with my son by my side.

One of my greatest sorrows is that life seems determined to sharpen us, making us all edges and hard lines. I don't blame us for that, not one bit, but I wish it wasn't so.

I have realised that even usually kind natures seem to carry ready thorns, pushed inwards in self-punishment, self-hate, or poised to prickle out in fear or bitter anger, in resentful defensiveness. How rare it is to find someone who is gentle through and through, in and out; gentle both to others *and* themselves, gentle in both their thoughts and in their reactions. How can gentleness be that difficult? It feels like it should be such an easy thing.

I have seen it in myself, time and time again, this instinct to clench and close off every time something goes awry. I feel it happen often even now, the many days my mind grows teeth.

I guess I'm learning the truth: that although we think of gentleness as an absence of aggression, perhaps it is the biggest fight of all. To harden, that's the easy road. But to soften, to choose always to melt into gentler, kinder thoughts, gentler acts, gentler living, while not losing sight of yourself, while remaining something solid and whole, something active and healthy in the middle, that's what takes a warrior's strength, isn't it? That's what takes the deepest resolve. And I so want to be that brave. I want to be that strong. I believe it is possible. I believe now that I can choose it, one redirected thought at a time.

Make peace. I say the words as I climb the stairs, as I say goodnight and turn off the light: you must make peace. It isn't ever going to be handed to me whole and solid, a brand-new house to step into and hide myself in forever more. I'm going to have to make it around me and even then, it will be something fragile. I will have to care for it and renew it, every day, patching it up and smoothing it out. Over and over, I shall just have to keep trying. Over and over to my heart, I shall say, 'Be soft, be soft, be soft.'

My son asleep, I sit on the sofa for a long while in the silence, and when my thoughts finally stop, I realise I can hear something. It is the dry crackle of a daffodil bud in its vase on top of the gas heater, slowly plumping itself to open, pushing against its paper casing to split it, ready to unfurl. Minutes go by and then I hear it again, the faintest rustle, little by little, push by push, until it grows still again, spent.

I can almost feel its gentle eagerness. How much is wrapped up in each bud. How tight and full it must feel, and I think: I know that feeling.

At least now I can say that I've been so quiet, I've heard a daffodil undress.

Spring

5.30 a.m. again. Sleep is something fragile lately. A robin is singing sweet and clear through the open bedroom window, and as I listen, I find I can hear the overlap of a blackbird too, but fainter, one territory over.

The different volumes give me a sudden feeling of distance. I can feel it between the sounds, that stretching of space. I realise these layers of song must exist again and again, each early bird taking up sound-space that overlaps another at its edges, like the way separate raindrops spread into each other on water. They must stretch the length and breadth of the island, these overlaid circles of sound, wakers like me rousing wearily in pockets of them, heads full.

That's how I will think of the dawn now: spreading, bird by bird.

★

THEN

The problem with telling a child what they're not is that it leaves a vacancy. It calls to someone else to take the job. To step in and tell you what you *are*.

His mother had died. She was sweet and smiling and he carried an echo of her face over his: dark, expressive, shining with something the rest of us lacked. It was a devastating, unfair death and he was right to be furious. Grief-stricken, his heart torn out, I believe he looked for something to fill the gaping, bloody maw of it. And there I was at twelve years old, hungry and blank, so he chose me.

The doctors had told me what my body was not – it wasn't something I should pay attention to. He, a year older, wanted to show me what it was really for, and because he seemed to know everything and needed me, I followed, willingly, not listening to anything my body said in response. I was just grateful for somewhere to go, something to do.

Of course, what we're told about our bodies affects our experience of sex. Intimacy, too. How could it not? There was always going to be a reckoning – many – it was just that the first for me came early.

The first time he kissed me in the dark cinema, his young, thick hands determined, eager, I went home and shook and wept in secret through the long night, devastated for reasons I didn't understand. It made a noise inside me so loud, so splitting, that I wasn't sure I could bear it, and yet I must have said yes again.

I was glad to be chosen, that's the truth of it. What did it matter now that I struggled to feel close to anyone at my new school, that I was awkward and defective? Now I had him. 'You're mine now' he'd tell me, intensely, dazzling, his face close to mine, and I would nod and smile and say, 'Yes, yes I am.' There was a safety in it, in thinking that I finally understood something about this life and my place in it.

He was always so sure, as if he'd been doing all this for years, but he couldn't have done: he was still only a child himself. I do remember that there were stories of an older girl before me. That is how it goes in your teens: touch is passed from one initiate to another, like gossip. Sometimes it is distorted badly, dangerously in the passing. That is how damage spreads too. Before long, all are infected, infectious.

He went to my church. He went to my new school. Soon there wasn't a day without him.

★

I watch the slow shuffle of another morning at the community centre. Forks are raised, papers turned, throats cleared. An old man sits across from me doing a crossword. I've not seen him here before. He wears a jumper the colour of old acorns and just-stirred gravy and has pulled the knitted collar up. Something about that jumper must have felt good when he saw it, as he carried it to the sales counter. Or perhaps it was wrapped carefully by a son who worried about his chest. This thought warms me. Either way, he picked it out when he dressed this morning, and now he sits, settled in front of me like a new day, tapping the point of his biro against the newspaper as he tries to fit letters to squares before committing.

I love the jumper and him: the pucker of it as it meets his comfortable belly, the slight shake of his hands under blue cuffs. Elbow patches hold him gently by the arm and I want to do the same. I want to whisper, 'You are loved', but I keep my seat, suddenly wary of my storytelling.

I look at the words I've scribbled about him on the page of my notebook. I know nothing about this man. I know very little about anyone here: where they've come from, where they're going next, the truth of what they carry or what they need. Some things they tell me, some things I am brave enough to ask, but for the most part, I am simply guessing. It weighs on me heavily today, how hard it is to know someone, how hard it is to know myself. There is such responsibility in all of it.

I have survived this life by shaking off the years and days or even hours before, like you'd shake yourself after a rainstorm. It all soon dries out and, here, I am too enamoured with some new sight, some new chance, to want to carry much with me. I have shallow pockets. I don't usually spend much time on remembering and I believe this is how it should be. It is a good way to endure. It is a lighter way to live.

And – oh – it's just, the view is too enticing. Who'd want to spend all their time in the wallow and suck of the past when there is the dry, bright land of now to be in? Where there is this and this and *this*? The younger man striding past me now, bouncing on his soles, flat cap like an arrow, his arm rising slowly as he moves to greet someone out of sight. Or the soft-faced lad at the café counter who pulls the zip of his fleece up a little higher around the blush of his acne, all youth and sweetness. By noticing and describing them in the here and now, it feels like I can sanctify them, love them, in my own shy way. It feels safe.

Writing about the past feels different. The truth is that I am frightened of it, of remembering, of piecing together older tales. Memory is fluid and capricious. I know things change down in the dark water of the past. I know they are hungry and have needs that are harder to meet. I tell myself that the clean-handed present just wants to be *seen,* noticed, and that feels easy enough, but the past demands to be understood. It makes history, remembering, a delicate pastime, bloated with assumption, with desire, and with things to prove. I know how much I could get wrong.

For years I refused to remember. Now, I tiptoe around my memories gingerly, wary of my interference, but I want to try, even though I know that memories are fragile, because I know now that it isn't enough to be only here and here and here again; not if we want to live well. What's more, whatever it feels like, the present doesn't exist unadulterated any more than my past does. The ground isn't firmer or more reliable when it comes to storytelling and observation. How easily I could reduce my self-assured, ever-present gaze to nothing but safe entertainment, designed to please or disappoint me, and call it good attention. How easy it would be for me to lose compassion, perspective, responsibility, to infantilise this old man in front of me, dressing him up in whimsy. We all do it, in our different ways. We create stories about people that have very little to do with them and everything to do with ourselves.

The more I write, read, watch, the more I learn. I learn that life is many things at once and that each moment is loaded. That we are all whole people carrying whole lives. Old programming shapes our days and how we view them, distorting how we see other people too. Our present shapes and reshapes our memories: nothing fixed, all fluid. I am learning that nothing exists as separate from anything else and that what comes before affects what comes after, hand to hand, all down the line. I am learning that despite it all, we can change.

I want to try and write it down, as honestly and as lovingly as I can. The past, the present: all of it. And I know that the work of seeing clearly begins with myself. Once I can see myself exactly as I am, no more or less, and see what made me, I can do the same to the world I live in. I can see where I stop and others begin. I can hold the man and his crossword a little more loosely and respectfully for that. I can scan my words for judgements and assumptions and look out for where my own story might try to overshadow his. Maybe then I can let him exist, all on his own, without getting in the way. Now that, that feels like love.

The larch tree waves outside the window. Fifty years before, perhaps its seed split at the same time the man tap-tapping his paper held up his own newborn child. Perhaps it didn't. I want to make space for their real histories, their future: for wild, changeable truths. I sit, legs burning, and remember a different child; one who was always afraid. I remember and wonder if my memories have changed since the last time I recalled them. I wonder what my mind has done with them, and why.

Slowly, I am learning to be braver. I think now I can hold what was past carefully, for just a little while. I can tell a story the best I can and honour it and the people within it. I can leave room to be wrong. I can move with time and remember that I am only ever, always, right here now. When I am frightened,

I can come back to safety and this slow, spring day, to the fresh green of the budding trees, to the rustle of the newspaper and the lad laughing as he serves the teas and all the other stories these things contain, and I can make room for them too. With this wider knowing, I can embrace the world whole.

The man stops to fold the crossword and shifts in his seat, catching my eye. His eyes are warm. I smile at him with everything I am in that quiet, strange moment – just one in an unfathomable chain – and he smiles right back.

★

THEN

The adults in our world thought it sweet: our holding hands, our public devotion to one another. Everyone seemed confident that this was what my body was for now, to be in the hand of this charming, tragic boy. 'Young love!' they'd exclaim as they saw us at church or in the street, and I'd feel reassured, unsure. His grieving father and my distracted parents were more cautious but seemed relieved that something good was happening – that he was happier and that I seemed better. I assumed they knew best. I assumed that they'd step in if there was any real danger.

The Bible classes we both went to some weekday evenings: they confused the matter in a different way. I'd sit on one of the padded chairs arranged in a circle and stare at the carpet, feeling his gaze on me. When you were that age, all the priests talked about was sex. They stressed how special it was, how sacred. Your virginity belonged to God, to your future husband, to anyone but you. A malignant thing to tell a girl desperate to please. A malignant thing to tell a girl who felt her body was wrong and in need of redemption; that she was a gift to be given away. He'd answer their questions confidently, piously, as if he had nothing to lose.

When he was upset, he'd break apart with rage. It happened often and without warning. He'd show me where he'd punched the wall, the door, show me the red mess of his knuckles. He'd show me calmly, without visible regret or sorrow. It felt like he might break apart at any moment, splinter like bone into something sharp and deadly. 'You're helping him so much,' I remember a voice saying. I thought it was my job to hold him together. I didn't know about warning signs back then. I knew about pain though. I could feel how much he hurt. I wanted to make it better.

I don't remember making a choice. There was no resolve, only a numb inevitability, a sense of good-natured duty. I'd lie awake after each step closer we made, closer to something that felt hot and treacherous, consumed with guilt, with shame, wondering if I was damned. But I couldn't feel God, however hard I tried, and this boy was real and he wanted me, needed me. 'We'll get married one day anyway,' he said, his hands on me, and mine on him now, and I believed him. I couldn't see beyond it. I couldn't see beyond anything.

He went to London to stay with some relatives, and I was allowed to go too. The flat was very white and full of books, the ceilings high, and it smelt of something adult and foreign, no trace of childhood anywhere. I think I knew in advance that it was going to happen then. It didn't occur to me that I could say no or if I would. I remember it hurt and my heart felt sick and I bled on the sheets again, but that was just my body and its noise. It was always making me feel horrible and I wasn't supposed to listen.

I do not remember other thought or feeling. It was simply a necessary procedure of devotion and care. I remember I couldn't speak the next day and shook, white and nauseous, till I got home. I was just unwell, I said, the new lie slipping as easily from me as everything else.

I was always unwell. No one thought anything of it.

★

I sit on the bench of one Mr Ray Archer, 1936–1995. His plaque invites me to 'Rest a While' and so I do.

My mobility scooter sits a little way away in the darkness of the yew tree. There is a blackbird in the conifers and my warmest brown boots have turned black with dew. There are three pairs of socks hidden underneath them and still my feet are cold, but it is good to be outside in the March air. The changing year is making me want to be, even if it's painful. Besides, a cemetery is a good place to be chilled and slow. No one will rush me here.

I read the names of my companions in short trips up and down the headstones, leaning balanced on two walking sticks, and then I come back to Ray to write. There must be a thousand lives here, more. I wonder if any of them ever met? Is there a past affair hidden in these respectable rows? An illegitimacy, a rivalry, a betrayal? I wonder what friendships and connections I could draw like lines between the stones. I imagine covering the whole graveyard in red wool stretched taut, pinned from one grave to another, marking which lives intersected others, joining everyone up again.

It is a small town, or it was, before the sprawling housing estates grew to eat the fields. The former residents lie grouped by family name, some squashed close, some determinedly apart. I imagine they lived that way too. This is not a wealthy community's graveyard. A good half of the cheap stones have collapsed in on themselves, scooped away by the rain. You'd struggle to find many legible dates over 100 years old, all melted away into sagging hollows.

On the ones I can still read, I see the same words over and over: *sleep, rest, thy will, beloved, memory, not forgotten, not forgotten*. It is our biggest fear, perhaps, to be forgotten, except many of these people will have been already. That is the way of things. I find a tiny, mossed-over, unkept gravestone with a name and a single faded date. The inscription reads: 'such a far-reaching loss for one so small' and I wonder how many ripples of that one child's loss are still spreading or whether he too has stilled for good. He touched me, at least, stirred me, and so endures a little longer.

All these past people. So many names, each one given in a moment to the baby they were once. The married names forever joined on one headstone move me. What did they give each other? How did they overlap and how were they separate? I imagine I can hear their pain and their joy like birdsong, rising off the stones.

I hear my first chaffinch of the year, and then a dunnock, robin, greenfinch, and imagine laughter, shouting, singing alongside them. I imagine lifetimes' worth of red-hot jealousy and black grief, and days that felt empty, all released into the air. I picture sparks of inspiration and connection fizzing from each life. Butterflies in stomachs, clenched fists, tender skin, desperate need. Everything I have ever felt will have been felt by someone here, sometime. I know this suddenly, with certainty.

Oh, it makes me dizzy. I wonder what they dreamed of, what their favourite thing to eat was. What did their best loved chair look like and where did they feel most at home? I wonder what gifts were given to them and which they treasured; if they ever read a book that made them cry. I wonder what they thought about in the dark and which conversations took more courage than they thought they had. I imagine them waiting. I imagine them bored. I imagine them feeling lesser to someone else in their life and the burn of it.

Does anyone else remember these things about them still? More importantly, did anyone notice these things about them when they were alive? Did they have an attentive observer? Someone to notice the way their mouth twisted when they were afraid, or how they always sat down to brush their teeth?

I hope they were noticed. If I could wish anything for them, I would wish for that.

The wind changes. It carries the smell of manure from a faraway field and suddenly death is here. We are so frail and yet we hold ourselves like stone in the world. Is that why we use it to mark our place? A last defiance against our true nature?

Lichen covers everything. It makes necklaces of powdered bone and teeth on the headstones, white, green and yellow. I peer at it through my magnifying glass and from above it looks, in turn, like a forest, like coral, like plague, like pus-covered skin, like chalk on a paving stone drawn by a child's hand. There is so much delight and horror everywhere, all at once, all the goddamn time.

A buzzard calls above me, its wings wide. Now that is how I would like to end: as feather and wing, not stone. That is what should happen when memory of you finally fades to nothing. Your stone should soften and, unfolding, the letters of you stretched in pattern, you should take to the sky.

When memory runs out, you should be released.

I think I would look forward to being forgotten then.

★

THEN

He'd point out places in scripture that said I belonged to him now. He'd laugh as he did so, in his neat polo shirts, because even he knew it was audacious to think that in this day and age. It felt like a lesson anyway.

He wanted to be a priest. Everyone said he had the making of one. Everyone told him he was special and his teenage hurt and insecurity must have gulped down the idea greedily. He could play the piano better than anyone I'd ever heard. A child genius – raw, natural talent, straight from God. It seemed to prove the case. I had been taught to serve God, and this boy who they heralded as a gift from Him became more and more muddled in my mind with that service. I sometimes wonder if it got muddled up in his mind, too.

He was lost, the hole in his heart hungrier, hungrier. 'Mine', he decided, meant more than my body now: it meant my obedience and faithfulness. He began to control what I wore, what I did, what I read. It was all training, he said, for being a good vicar's wife.

He decided I shouldn't talk to anyone but him, to prove how much I loved him. He would say it with a warning scowl. I was obedient and began to say only the most necessary words. I began to think only the most necessary thoughts, too.

Time passed. I don't know how long it was. I think I stopped dreaming then. Perhaps that is why my memories of that time are so disjointed and so strangely spaced apart. There is static when I think I stopped existing at all. To look back is like turning a dial on a radio, all dark with these flashes tuned in, loud and jarring. What friends I had, already distanced by my many times of separation, wandered away for good, disgusted. They didn't like him, so they didn't like me either. There was another short hospital stay for more nerve blocks to my lower legs but I remember little of it. I remember he hated it, that's all. It was harder to control who I talked to in there.

The girls around me all tried to dress like one or other of the Spice Girls, or they rebelled and wore Nirvana t-shirts and combat trousers and dyed their hair black. I did none of these things, agreeing to the sedate dresses he picked, the tops that wouldn't reveal any cleavage, not that I had any. At school, the other kids laughed at my ankle socks, my thick glasses. 'Good,' he'd say. 'I don't want anyone else looking at you. Don't take your jumper off today. You can see your bra through that shirt.'

I sweated in my seat and tried not to look up.

★

I always forget what this feels like, this spring fever, this new light.

There is a rising in me. My hands and my lips have become hungry buds and I want to press them against whatever's warm and giving. I *feel* it: that sap pulse, an awakening of green somewhere hidden and parched. It is like nothing else.

Everything around me is remembering how to be itself again. My garden is only small: a few metres long, barely two wide, and yet I have filled it over the years, slowly lining the edges with raised flowerbeds, prising back paving slabs to find soil. Now, the bleeding heart by the wall has pushed up red fingers that collect the dew. The rose bushes, clematis, and honeysuckle have begun to pin ruffled rosettes to their chests, announcing their names. There is an imperceptible narrowing of the gaps between the distant trees as their branches bare tiny new fists. I cannot help but reach out to touch it all, the fleshy whirl of future tulip, allium, a fingertip placed gently to every sign of low, green regrowth. 'I remember you,' I say, smiling at everything in affirmation.

Every year, I think my world dead and then grow giddy at its renewal. I glide, punch drunk, on the first truly bright March days, face to the sky, and feel like I could stretch into it until I scatter.

All around me, things are finding their place, their wings, their voice. There are daisies in the verge again – *daisies!* Giant queen bumblebees split the air like juggernauts; starlings call their swanee whistle greetings like cheerful bombs dropping, and the trill of the smaller birds, sparrow and finch and tit, dunnock and wren, overlap until every last second is full to overflowing.

I want to eat it whole. I want to swallow the lot and let it continue inside me: a fat, green goddess. Winter is forgiven in a heartbeat.

A robin lands a foot from my left ear. I stop dead, eyes closed, and for half a perfect minute there is nothing but his song, his hope, his ferocity.

Once again, another year older, I cannot for the life of me comprehend how it is possible for a world to feel this alive.

★

THEN

He'd find ways to check, to make sure of me. I'd look up from my lesson and see him, framed by the square window of the classroom door, beetroot red and furious, incandescent, a dark promise in his face. The classroom doors all had those square windows and so nowhere was safe. The worst days of all were when I was caught sat by another boy, even if I'd had no choice. I remember long afternoons of waiting for the fallout, numb with dread, the voices around me muffled, meaningless.

Punishment was quick and brutal, childish, hidden. I don't remember the first time. He'd spit in my face. My arms would be squeezed into bruises, simply, harshly. He'd push my glasses into my face with his palm until my eyes ran and I saw stars. My legs, still regularly full enough of their pain to make me limp and need a stick or crutches some days, were an easy target. He'd kick them, just once, sharp with his thick-soled shoes and I'd feel it spread up my legs into my spine. I remember the greying cuffs of his white school shirts and how they'd yellow under the arms. I remember the smell of sweat and TCP. I remember ribs that ached for weeks.

I never fought back. I simply crumpled, leaking tears and pleading apologies, defeated, pitiful. I was already not talking about how I felt. It was easy to not talk about this too.

And yet, I was always so shocked when it happened again. I remember incredulous horror. I remember his blue inhalers and the noise his chest made as he wheezed. If I had been bad, he would refuse to use them in front of me, wordless, gasping, purple. He'd tell me of all the pills he was going to take. All was clear: this was my fault. I begged for forgiveness. I begged him not to die. I was convinced that if I took one more step wrong, he would.

I made it easy because I adored him. I adored him and I was more frightened of him than anyone I have ever known since. I needed him desperately. I would weep at his absence, terrified, because the fear of what would come next, of what he might be thinking in the interim, was worse than anything else. And he could be kind too, wonderfully kind and soft and generous. To be with him when he was happy was heaven because it didn't contain all the bad things I feared the rest of the time. The evenings we were apart, I wrote ardent letters full of promises so he'd know I'd done nothing but sit and think of him. I was sure they would keep me safe.

When he was happy, I felt I'd achieved something. How easy it was to mistake relief for my own happiness and comply with it all one more time.

★

I can't get anything to go right today. It is taking me too long to move from room to room. The day races on beyond my capacity, mean and unstoppable, not pausing for a minute to let me catch up. My son races with it to go and fetch an extra walking stick from the basket as I shuffle. I try not to look at the clock. Tea is late and I don't know what to make. I end up heating baked beans in the microwave again. 'Oh, I don't mind, Mummy,' he says.

I can feel it, the pulse of an old refrain. Useless. Hopeless.

Not for the first time, I realise I am holding a funeral for power and independence in my head as I try to move. I'm singing dirges as if it's all gone, all lost, and I'll never get it back. The mourning song overlays the late sun through the window and the babble of my bright son as he talks about his day.

Stop. I know better than to do this now. I know that even if I feel like so much resigned, dead wood, that if I pare myself back carefully enough, patiently enough, I will always find green, sap-rich life. Or if not green, an ember. Find it and I can blow on it gently, care for it and nurture it, and no one can take it from me. Remember, Jo. Remember.

I stop and watch the split of narcissus bulbs in the planters on the windowsills where a month ago there was only bare earth. I reach for my boy's hand, to stroke it gently, the way he loves, as we make our way back to the sofa together, unwrapping his thoughts as we go. 'I was sure I heard a humpback whale at school today, Mummy. I'm SURE of it. ALSO, did you know that the long-armed squid is the only squid with elbows?' I start to smile through his chatter. I let it fill me.

I want him to know this power too, to know that he can raise his thoughts and his words and his breath. That he can always choose, even if only to reach an inch forward. Neither of us will ever be in a place or a time when all choice and light is gone forever. The force of that makes my fist clench, my grin widen, my teeth show.

I carry power inside of me. I carry it hot and ripe. I need only point my will and move, infinitesimally slow and ordinary but forward. It doesn't need to be dramatic or impressive. No one need see it but me and him, as we hang the laundry together, as I pull the plug on the dirty dishwasher, as we decide to watch nature programmes on my laptop in my bed.

Power is given and taken, but not all of it. Never all of it.

I let myself feel it again as we lie close together in the dark: that tiny power spark.

'See?' it says, 'I'm still here. Not lost. Not dead.'

★

THEN

I don't remember much else. I don't remember my parents, where they were, what they said, what they did. I had obediently cut all lifeboats adrift, them included. I remember missing them, missing feeling close to them, to something. I remember them telling me to keep the door open a crack when he was over, but I simply learnt to be quieter.

Two, three years it went on for. Years lost to static, until one day it was over, just like that. I was fifteen and I told him that I didn't want to be with him any more. I remember feeling the courage in me like a furnace, chest straining like it might rip, but I don't remember where it came from or how it grew. He threw an ornament at me: a heavy, oversized rabbit that sat on the floor of my bedroom. I dodged and it hit the wall by my head. My dad took him home. I'd often put my fingers to the dent it left afterwards, next to the white sailboat that I had thought would keep me safe. There was nothing else left to look at, nothing to examine to help me understand it all. Only that hollow in the wall and a shame I couldn't shake.

I carried the guilt of it for a long time. I would tell myself that if I'd been brave enough to shout out once, maybe both of us could have been saved, but I was silent, mouth simply opening and closing again, drowning as I was, and I did nothing. I didn't know how.

It has taken me a long time to understand power, control, trauma: his and mine. It has taken me a long time to understand fear.

I do not hate him. It is long gone. You do not have to forgive the people who hurt you, but when the power grew in me to make real, informed choices of my own, that is one I chose. I let my pain see his. He was a product of what had come before, as was I. There was an after for him too, his own story. I wish him peace sometimes, when I think of him. I wish him peace in the after.

Real stories never conclude, they only continue. And so, we go on.

I didn't go to church again.

★

He comes to me quietly, curtains closed, all shadow.

'Mummy?'

I swim through the last vestiges of sleep to find him. It is early. I gather his dark shape into my arms with a mumbled good morning and he finds his best fit, folding over on top of the duvet across my chest. His head meets its familiar place at my collarbone, his glasses digging in just a little. He says nothing for three long beats. It is enough time for my fingers to find the twist of hair that bunches at the back of his neck and for me to take in a full breath of him, his weight pulling gently at my lungs.

'Do you know my favourite kind of picture?' he asks, suddenly loud and sitting upright. I cannot see his face clearly in the dim room.

'I don't,' I reply, and the words catch thick in my unused mouth. I cough to smooth them. 'What is your favourite kind of picture?'

He shifts to pull his hands from where he'd tucked them under me and raises them, a conductor in his dressing gown getting ready for something important.

'It's when you have, like, a shape,' he says, 'a dark shape, and light coming here.' He gestures, and I see the shadow of him frown in concentration. 'But *this* is black and, and, around it is light.' He stumbles with the words, stuck, and drops his hands, defeated.

'Do you mean like a silhouette?' I say, gently, and his whole body moves with his affirmation.

'Yes! Yes, that's what I mean.' His back is straight and eager now and I can feel the energy in him already, the day not even begun.

'Are you thinking of a specific picture? One you've seen?' I ask.

A headshake. 'No, it's just . . . I can see what I mean, in my head. Like a city skyline?

I nod and smile, not sure if he can see me.

Three more beats while we both think of his picture. I smile again in the dark at the shape he is making in the half-open door, silhouette himself in the light cast from the bathroom window down the hall.

'You can make those kind of pictures with a camera, you know, if you look where the light is coming from,' I say, inspired, and feel his fingers find my hands, pushing their way into them as I speak, needing connection. 'So, if you had someone standing here, and you noticed that the light was coming from behind them, from the sun, or from a window if you're inside . . .' It is my turn now to pull my hands away to help me, and I shift my shoulders up the pillows to let me gesture better. 'And then you stood *here*, in front of them, and took a photo, you'd get their silhouette.'

'Yes!' He gets it. 'Like if . . . like if the cat was to sit on the radiator by your window, and you took a photo of him?'

I grin wider. 'That's it! And then if you were to change it and have the light behind YOU—'

He interrupts. 'Like you're in the shadow and the light is over *there* by the person,' he says it again, still stuck on his image, not hearing me. 'Light here and dark here . . .' His busy hands are moving again too.

'That's right, then you'd have a silhouette photo. But if you moved and stood where the light is, with it behind you,' I try again, forever a mother with a desire to teach, 'the dark behind the other person, then the light will shine on them and you'll get a super clear photo. That's how you get a lovely, bright image.'

'Yeah!' He smiles. It is lighter in here already. The freckle on his top lip is visible: my favourite one. 'Mummy, can I watch TV?'

He's up and moving even as he says it and I laugh a yes, my chest and my bed empty again, my heart full. I am left to hear the thunder of the stairs and to stretch and wake more slowly.

★

THEN

I crouched on the porch step and held her long, shining hair away from her face as she vomited weakly into her parents' front border. It was her sixteenth birthday, a full six months ahead of my own, and all inside were already clumsy with cheap booze.

I didn't know her well. She was one of the popular girls, bemused by me but friendly enough. I had obligingly gone halves on a bottle of peach schnapps obtained from somewhere and tried to look as if I was enjoying myself. I never really did at these events that were somehow secretly part of my life now, but that was my abnormality, not theirs, I was sure of that, and so I played along, grateful for the invitation.

The kitchen lights were too bright, the laughter too loud. I drank until things span just a little and I stopped looking sober, completing my disguise. At that point, everyone else stopped noticing if you were drinking or even saying anything at all, and so I stopped doing both, relieved.

Freedom had turned out to be confusing, terrifying and sublime. I want to write that I burst into it, opening, becoming something clean and beautiful, but I didn't. I dripped out into my new life apologetically, like thick primordial soup.

The business of friends was most urgent and so I did my best to make people like me again. I wasn't very good at it, but my oldest friend from primary school who had ended up at my high school drew me back into her circles. I fidgeted on the edge of them and tried not to embarrass her. The boys in my year had written me off as pathetic and not to be taken seriously and so mostly ignored me. The girls were kinder and more forgiving, although some would still talk to me with a gleam in their eyes and a tilt to their heads. I would doubt their words and not know what to say. It made it hard to see them as anything other

than predators. It made it hard to relax. I know now
that they will have been full of their own fears, but
I didn't know that, then.

My mum and dad did their best to listen to my
guarded words and permit me the independence
I asked for, but there was a gap between us now and
I couldn't seem to close it. I hadn't told them much
about what had happened, before. I didn't tell them
about what was happening now. I didn't really know
how to talk to them, to anyone.

There were boys at this party, clever and cruel,
and I was even more nervous than usual, so it was a
reprieve to be the one to go outside and hold hair
back, even though I shook with cold. I remember the
shaking, wearing the wrong clothes, my breath visible
under the dark sky and the porch lamp. I remember
that I could see the stars. I was still very afraid, after all
that business with the boy.

That's how I'd think of it: 'that business'. Past. Done.
I didn't want to talk about it anyway.

★

I've got a thing about overhead wires. I can see
some from every window in my house. I like the
spaces between them, like someone's cut up the sky
and pieced it back. I like the way they stretch from
house to house, the fact that we're all joined up like
that: threaded together.

Today, I want to attach paper cups to the ends of them and shout. I want to tug at them and see if someone at the other end tugs back. I want to flick them and watch them bounce and startle the starlings, or use them like catapults to fire water balloons a mile or more. I want to run along them feeling the tension and release in my bare soles. I reckon I could cross the whole country like that. I'd go and see who sits at the other ends of them because I am lonely again today.

My one complaint is that they're only black or silver. I want colours. You could pick yours and I could pick mine and we'd crisscross the town like May revellers.

I expect they'll be gone one day. We'll find a more sophisticated, more hidden way of doing things and I will miss them. We need more reminders that we're all attached, I think, not fewer. I worry we're forgetting.

★

THEN

It felt momentous that I was to turn sixteen soon. I had been convinced that I would be ready by now: finished. I looked at the reality, horrified.

The word 'potential' was still passed around, over my head at parents' evenings, pulsing from school reports. Now I knew it was the right word for me because I wasn't anything good, not yet. I had used to be. I would think back to my early years and remember a sense of something light and confident, a knowing, a wholeness, but I had been unmade since then. I had been careless and lost myself.

I didn't know for a long time that becoming was about paring yourself back, about deep listening to something quiet and truthful, undramatic and vulnerable – I thought it was about *addition*, about covering all of that up. I tried to make the sum of me as big and impressive as I could, to hold a shape around me to hide my own, and felt despair at the constant slippage. I begged my parents for money to buy clothes that the other girls wore – first from Top Shop, then from loud Birmingham markets when my friends decided grunge was cooler. I tagged along to sit in the bedrooms of boys with heavy fringes who played guitar and still frightened me. I picked up their CDs and asked if I could borrow them to copy, and when they asked me what I thought of them, I'd run out the practised words and judgements that I'd heard other people using, hoping I hadn't got it wrong. I plastered on some shape of personality and hoped it would solidify, eventually, into something real. I was sure that underneath I was nothing. I was determined that no one would find out.

In lessons, I'd sit and feel under the tables for the hard, round fossils of chewing gum, years old, reassured by them. They spoke of others who had sat in this spot and grown on. I wondered how they'd managed to survive.

I assumed survival was inevitable. It's funny: despite it all, I've always assumed that.

★

I spent long months craving this escape and now I'm here, I don't know what to do with myself.

'Here' is a lodge with my son, my mum, her partner and my brother, for a few days in a holiday park on the edge of a lake in Derbyshire, under bare alder tree and pine. If you run a finger along any branch, you loosen a rainshower. There was snowfall at the weekend, the April kind: warm, wet and brief. In the thaw, all is muted brown, green and grey. All is perfect. I can hardly bear to look directly at it. It has been a year since I left the house for any extended length of time.

It has made me even quieter than usual. The footpaths run with loud, unfamiliar faces. I find I want to stay close to the house even though we have hired a mobility scooter for me to use here and my wheelchair is in the car. I retreat to corners to watch and test my place in things. I keep my gaze low, looking up and out at the overlap of branches that cradle the lodge only sometimes, after a deep breath.

I don't know why I feel so small and vulnerable, but I do. I feel like I must keep myself held in, so I don't give myself away. It feels pathetic to describe it so, but there it is.

I think maybe I have grown used to safe silence, to sparse beauty that is sought out and peeked at, not this abundance of it. I have grown used to solitude. I have learnt to temper my sensory overwhelm by steering clear of 'too much', and this last winter was obliging in its restriction. Here, I am dazzled and noise-numbed, jumping at every cupboard bang and companionable bustle, even here in the lodge with the loving family I have known all my life. I smile through it, but something in me is all flinch.

I find I need to be outside and alone whenever possible. When the others are happy and busy, I have taken to dragging a patio chair a few steps away from the house, leaning on it as I go like a walker, step by step through the muddy ground, until I am out and under the trees.

From this place, there is nothing in my line of sight but bark and water, the public paths hidden and distant. The wildlife is abundant. Pink-footed geese and their Canadian cousins share the grass with almost-grown cygnets. Ducks snooze while coots and moorhens pick around them. There is always a squirrel on the patio table and a pair of chaffinches flitting from fence to floor. We are watched over by rock doves, huddled in the trees.

It is the rabbits I love best. They live in the lake bank and have learnt a boldness. Soon, they are lolloping around my feet and this last time that I pull up the chair to sit, finally something in me begins to loosen. I have been sad, I realise. Sad and disappointed in myself. I wanted to embrace all this, rare as it is. I wanted to do better. To do *more*, to *give* more – oh I don't know, but now I'm here, I can't. I try to love the things and people around me the best I can, but here I can only hunch and watch. I am trying to understand why.

One rabbit stops to wash itself, paws pulled rhythmically over nose and head. I am tempted to copy, to pull at my ears until they stretch, to crouch till I shrink, and finally, in the form I belong in, to burrow into the dark home of the bank and find soft, congruous fur against my flank, quiet heartbeats, pink tongues. I think then I would feel all right.

I so rarely know how to be acceptable; how to be unwild. We love to talk of being wild in human terms – as something exciting, alluring, the stuff of movies and pin-ups – but when you watch wild things, you begin to understand that this is not what wildness means. It is nothing so conveniently pleasing.

To be truly wild is to be skittish, capricious, trusting of few. It is to be pulled to home and warmth and the sensory comfort of familiar bodies, not to newness and excitement. To be wild is to be wary, heeding instinct louder than promise. It is the hope that those who see you will see you only for love, not as prey, and a wish for not too many eyes on you at once. It is to crave simplicity: an undisturbed spot, a full belly, a body that knows itself. To be wild is to be drawn to sing one perfect song over and over, like the great tit in the pine trees now, and for that to be enough for you to belong where you are.

It is to live close to death and change but not let it panic you into worse. It is to steer yourself endlessly towards the things that nurture you, to be unable to stop or deny yourself.

I am wild. This is why I struggle here, struggle a little everywhere that does not fully feel like home. Out here amongst the other wild things there is some comfort in that.

It is night now. In a moment, I will go to bed and lie down in the dark beside the sleeping shape of my son in our shared room and I will feel right again. Maybe I can enjoy this place in my own, wild way. I may not be able to manage the rakish, feel-good kind of being that seems most valued here and everywhere, but if I tried to pick up a rabbit, I bet it would bite.

It knows itself and its limits. It trusts them, and I should trust mine.

★

THEN

I was well enough to say yes to things, anything – a rare thing in my life – and I thought that was living, and so I said it over and over: yes, yes, yes.

I started to spend regular evenings at local bars and rock clubs. Nobody there seemed to care if you were underage, but we worked on our impression of sardonic, cocksure university students just to make sure. I remember endless eye-roving hours seeking out quieter spaces to sit down in, the speaker noise thrumming against the crouched and frightened truth of me. Each day, I tried to set my face, my hair, my body, into something vaguely acceptable, maybe even desirable if I was lucky, because like everyone else around me, I thought that someone desiring you was proof that you were doing OK. I skipped meals. Older men sidled up to me to ask what I was studying, and I lied. 'How old are you?' they'd ask, and I'd lie again. I played the game and convinced myself the reality wasn't obvious, but of course it was. We all knew our parts in the game. We all knew the script.

I had long ago learnt how to look like all was fine. Inside, I was a rigid blizzard. I'd hold it in until I could be alone. Only then could I shut down, lying awake with a dull, cold pulse, the evening still trapped inside of me. I spent much time exhausted and recovering, or trying to. I was always trying to find my feet again.

My memories smell of spilled beer. I can still feel the pull in my gut towards a boy my own age who I liked, tentatively, and who couldn't stand the sight of me. I can still hear the static of trying to work out the rules of all this. I would try to sit in the right place, in the right way, so I could be seen by him doing the right things. A laugh, a glance. I'd try to time my visits to the bathroom, to the bar, plan my route through the room. Then I'd go home drained, confused, my whole body a slumped tinnitus, wondering if it was like this for everyone, worried it was not.

Streetlights made a roving line in my vision through the windows of the bus on my way home. I'd watch them rise and fall, soothed by their rhythm, their consistency. It never occurred to me that the answer lay in soft things, not in noise.

★

Jude's house is the fourth place I spend time in. There is home, school, the community centre, and Jude's. They form a small rectangle on the map, less than a quarter mile long. They make up my world these last few years. Today we are together at her drafty old house on the main road, with its porch full of wellington boots and a vast pear tree in the garden. We'd planned to work, but everything we have to say since the last time we saw each other keeps us well distracted. Our pens and books lie discarded. We sit either side of her long dining table in the kitchen, my feet on the stool her youngest son uses to reach the counter and that I remember her elder two children using before that.

I haven't seen a soul all week apart from my own son. I swing between feeling elated and overwhelmed in her company, but I know she will understand that – she always does.

Some families you're born into, others you make, but another kind still is the family you find. I'm not even sure how it happens. There's no spoken consensus; no marriage or birth or ceremony, it's just that's what you are now. From the outside, no one would know it, no one would know to place you all together, but if they were to dig deep under the ground of you, they would see it: you're all joined up.

A few years ago, that's how I gained Jude. It was an inexplicable magic. We'd seen each other before, but a chance meeting at the small, glass-strewn playground between our houses one grey afternoon led to a conversation, then an invitation, then another. Me! Who'd never managed the back and forth of friendship well and who'd always had it go wrong; who'd long ago retreated into the safety of long-distance, sporadic acquaintances: I had a friend. A best friend.

I was surprised to feel so safe, so unclosed. It had been a long time since I last felt that. And over the years, we found we grew together. We found we grew *better* together. She didn't go away when things got rough, and neither did I. She didn't get scared in that way, or resentful, or irritated, and I didn't either. With her – my new sister – came brother-in-law, niece, nephews. I don't get to call them those things, not out loud, but that's what they are.

Jude speaks and a loose block of fringe falls from her face and curtains her oversized glasses. She tucks it back and talks some more. She has started a social enterprise designed to support women in our community and her passion shines from her, from the way she moves her hands, to the coloured Post-it Notes she sticks in her notebooks. I rarely notice her blinking, she always seems so awake, and yet she is often tired, and doubtful too, and there is good company in that, especially as she admits it. She doesn't know whether she's getting it right, all this. She doesn't know if any of this will do any good. We talk again, as we often do, about the power of small, slow, unseen things, reassuring each other. Again her fringe falls, and again she pushes it back, over and over. She has dropped many things this morning: her phone, her pen, her fringe, and patiently she has tucked and retrieved and carried on.

She lets my awkward words and laughter find a way out while I blush and feel a little panicked. In return, I listen to her search through her choices and possibilities. I try to leave space for her to explore her own, fierce mind. Each of us knows what sits in the room with us. She has her own worries and cares. We share our lot between us.

She has seen me at my very worst and there is no going back from that. She has kept pace with me as I've pulled myself across dirty floors, making me laugh through every painful inch. She has sat with me, firm and fierce and loyal as iron through benefit assessments, doctors' appointments, as I described the most embarrassing realties of my life only to cry with me as soon as the door was closed. She is the kindest, cleverest, funniest woman I have ever known and the closest friend I've ever had. Long months go by when she's the only one I see. I know, like I know the sky is blue, that she will be with me for life.

There is no sound but the eager slide of my highlighter pen across my book's page as we settle into silence again for the dozenth time. 'Ha!' she says. 'I love it when I can hear your highlighting getting faster and faster. I know you're happy then.' I hear the scrape of her underlining something in her diary in a companionable echo. I feel a warmth that sustains and never diminishes. In another hour we will pick the children up from school and they will all come running through the door and play and fight like siblings until it's time for tea.

We're taught that only romance can give us the love stories we crave. I say, come sit with me at my best friend's table one teatime, our formed-family delighting in every part of each other, my sister's eyes catching mine in love, in belonging at last, all of us laughing loud enough to make the sugar shake, and tell me you still believe that.

★

THEN

One day, a dawn broke and I did not notice. I opened a book of Georgia O'Keeffe paintings in an abandoned art classroom: a huge book that took two hands and a heave to lift it onto the scratched table. The colour, the movement, as I turned the pages made my mouth wet. I'd come back at lunchtimes to look again. I'd touch my fingers to the lines and the folds, and want to lick them after. I felt I was seeing flowers for the first time, seeing everything for the first time.

This is how life should be looked at, close up, like this, I'd think. This is how everything should be understood, loved. Part of me knew these pictures contained something secret, too: a key, a code, to some part of me, something adult, something powerful. I wanted it.

Soon after, I begin to copy her paintings, blending with my fingers: acrylic, pastel, charcoal. My touch

on the paper felt good. I begin to start looking down
the lens of a camera too, everything contained in a
neat rectangle. I'd shift it from place to place, looking,
scared to press the shutter, scared to get it wrong,
until with a gathering of courage, I'd press, I'd mark.

There began to be a rightness, at last. Still hidden,
still small, but something. Mine.

★

You can hear it, that point in the year. There is a
sound like a warm curtain opening and something
parts in front of you. It is velvet and ripe. You must
enter – you *must*.

I have done too much again. I couldn't help myself.
There has been a run of perfect April days, cool and
green and bright. When I close my eyes, I know that
the roses in my garden will be red-veined and ardent
in the sunshine, unfurling bloody new leaves against
the wallflowers. I know because I saw them like this
while I did too much; while I held them, loved them.

I sat and cut last year's dead loose, my legs sprawled
on the dirty floor as I reached and turned to pull the
pots towards me. I wished I could cut myself loose too,
just for a while, so I could rise to buzz and hover over
each thing there, round and matronly, and see what
was needed. I couldn't fight the temptation then, to
pull myself to standing and sway, fragile in the spring
air like a seedling myself. I couldn't help the joy of it.

Seeing a task waiting, I'd think, I could just do that one thing, couldn't I? I could just *try*? And that is why I lie here now, watching the new days from a distance, my body spent, mud still under my fingernails, my hair unwashed. I lie completely still, because that is the only thing for it, and I wonder what to do next.

Being someone who rests in a world that glorifies, fetishises work more than any other thing is to be an alien among your own kind. It is to be treated much like one, too. I must rest every day, most of the day. It is the only way for me to stay close to any kind of wellness. I have never been able to work a full-time job and it's been over a decade since I was able to work outside the house at all. This has meant reliance on state benefits, often – its own traumatic, impossible restriction – but there has been very little choice in that.

Each day, I sit removed from the world at work and it watches me, suspicious, assessing and resentful. I have learnt to watch it back. I have been in a good place to notice how not all work is good work, although we treat it as if it is.

Here, I have seen what overwork does to people, to families, to communities. I have realised that it doesn't count as 'productive' if you damage a whole lot of other things in the process. I have seen how work can be a form of self-harm, a form of sabotage, a form of avoidance and panic and dysfunction. It can be narcissistic and greedy, whatever the righteous façade.

Now, I know that just because someone is working, their work does not automatically get to be good or worthy of admiration. It's not that simple. It is a useful lesson to hold close after a lifetime of being told that hard work will cure me. The knottier lesson for me has been learning that all of this is true of rest too. There is wrong work, and there is wrong rest: the kind of rest that isn't rest at all, but simply a numb stupor we embrace when we don't want to face our life or feel anything at all. The kind that is sickly ripe and made for unhealthy consuming as we shovel our minds and hearts full of things that will not bring us peace or healing. I know this because I have spent too long reaching for things that numb in order to make life feel more bearable and calling it rest, but it has never helped, or not for long. It has never done anything other than rob me of better.

This then is my challenge: not to avoid work and its risks entirely or to fetishise it, but to embrace my potential for gentle action, slow change whenever I can. Not to rest, for rest I must, but to rest *well*.

Today, while my son is at school, I read, I write a little. I try not to pick up the numbing drug of my phone. I try not to think of work or rest at all. Instead, I ask, without judgement, what's happening right now? And what is the best thing to do next?

Right now, maybe, I think the answer is to lie very still and watch the light through the window. Later, it will be to take a deep breath and face the pummel of the trip to school and back. Tomorrow, to stop making excuses and to write until the writing is done. Yesterday, it was to play in the garden. I know that to choose well, I must only keep paying attention. I must be wide awake and brave, know what matters to me, and adapt to each moment. I must learn how to hold fast in a system that will always tell me that I'm *not enough*, whatever I do.

I believe in gentle, creative, practical action now above all else: conscious, malleable, chosen. Action not to prove my worth or meet anyone's expectations, but an unseen, calm momentum. Action that looks life straight in the eye.

There is room for grief here. Room for loss, for pain, for the pervasive disappointment that my happy hour in the garden has left me here, for the secret whisper of 'not fair'. There is room for everything. There's no need to ignore how I feel, I must simply try and act from this place the best I can, and then act and act again. I can always keep turning towards something, like the sweet pea seedlings on my windowsill whose elongated, wiry bodies stretch and shift as I turn them, reaching for the light. It can be the smallest shift, but still, I move.

I watch the lime tree through the square of glass and the shifting, blue sky. I know that by joining them, by committing to an active life, however unhurried, I join a dance with everything. I move carefully and joyfully and all moves with me. Some days, I want to shout it out of my open door. I am not one of the dead or inanimate lost, cold and numb! I am not dead, you hear me? I am never left behind, however much it might feel like it, however cruelly you might insist. I move through my day, pulling lightly on strings of cause and effect, and in that I can know myself meaningful in the middle of it. There is so much room for love, for gratitude, for celebration.

I lift my drink. I notice that the spider plant on the shelf is drooping, pour my glass of water around its roots instead, and go to fetch another, slowly, letting my muscles soften. I make my way to my son's room and fold t-shirts there until my legs shake, and then head back to bed. My small actions are how I can care for myself, for others, for my environment. And there is such power in knowing that every step I take can shape or change something, even if it is only myself and the solitary hours of my day, even if it is only in five-minute, ten-minute, determined, wilful bursts.

Now try and tell me that my life is lazy. Now look closer at my restful life and show me where I'm less than you, less than anyone.

I will tell you the best reason to live like this: there is no regret. Each new, rich and loving choice leaves it further and further behind.

★

THEN

I had taken an office job at a double-glazing firm. After school and on Saturday mornings, I'd sit in the empty back office and type invoices and letters on the boxy word processor.

There were times when I was happier there than anywhere else. I'd count down to the school bell and try to cadge a lift with a passing sixth-former so I could clock in half an hour early. I'd let myself in, call to the fitters in the workshop, and climb up the dark, narrow back stairs with their thin, scratchy carpet, feeling the ache in my legs after the day's lessons, breathing in the smell of damp in the walls.

I liked the always empty small showroom downstairs, full of leaded, coloured glass that caught the light in shifting patterns. I would sit in it when it was time to take a break. I'd wash stained, mismatched mugs in the workshop kitchen and make drinks for the brash window fitters, grouping them on the counter to requests of tea, coffee, milk, sugar, as they sang in sudden, tuneless bursts to the radio. I loved

them: their rough language, their swagger, their
cheerful care. The manager upstairs would smile and
talk to me sometimes in a way that pulled me in like
a tide. I thought him very handsome and felt a heat
in me around him, until some spell would break, and
he'd say, too loudly, 'Oh god, you're only sixteen,
aren't you? I forget. I forget', and he'd put his red face
in his hands, laughing.

I was paid cash in square brown envelopes. There
was little money to go around at home and I wanted
some of my own. I opened a bank account and paid
it in, renting a small television for my bedroom. I'd
watch old movies on video when I couldn't sleep.
The black and white pulse of the figures felt more
like sleep than real sleep, and I began to sense what
adulthood might be like on the other side of all this.

I began to think I might enjoy it.

★

There is a type of loneliness that fits perfectly with
heavy rain and an open window and climbing back
into your Saturday bed with coffee and an ache. With
all these things aligned, none of it needs fixing, not the
rain or the loneliness or the inactivity, or the pull that
rests somewhere between your heart and your thighs.

All get to thrum together comfortably with the
kind of intensity that feels like being held, despite
everything. And when the rain increases in a slow

crescendo, when the volume switch is turned, it is like the rise of a kiss, and my breath catches just the same, just the same.

★

THEN

Falling between the bruises and the clamour, there began to come flickers like these – the roving lights, the O'Keeffe book, my independent, solitary work. Flickers of becoming, of home and happiness. Not shaped yet, not discernible, but foreshadowings: the softest breath of exposure. The light that was to one day bring me back to myself found imperceptible footholds. It kindled small parts of me.

I would look in the mirror in the early morning, dim blue, and smile my practised smile: careful, mouth closed. My hair had always been shoulder length, difficult, thick, but I had begun to cut it shorter, and then shorter still, shorter than anyone else's. Rightness again; a click when all else in me hadn't fit. I dyed it bold colours, purple, red, black – the colours of Georgia's flowers – and in that there was a deeper exhalation; a sometimes, fragile loosening to that tight smile, as I finally began to like the person I saw.

★

I am watching the sun move around the garden. In early May, it claims its territory like a new lover. Here, it asks? And here? The light is soft, slow, perfect. By summer, all shyness will be lost as it wakes and slides in like a long-agreed promise. But for now, just now, I am enjoying these gentler beginnings. The garden smells of the last of the pink hyacinths and paperwhites, sweet and heavy with that undercurrent of secret decay. I am restless and cannot stay in my seat for long.

The truth is that no one has touched me for a while. Not in the way you know I mean. Not in the way that gives you something rather than taking away.

What touch there has been in the last few years has been complicated, anxious, sporadic. Pain makes touch disorientating, the overlapping sensations competing until it is hard to feel anything but panic. Sex has only happened occasionally, often with regret in the afterthought, and it has not been chosen wisely. My desire got caught up in my slowly worsening mobility, my confusion, my grief. Loneliness can make us fools so often; grief too. In the end the shame got too much, and I simply avoided it altogether.

But, with the spring there comes a languid, quiet remembering. I have a knowing body; an ageing body that is beginning to stop apologising for itself. One that has begun to stop needing the reassurance of youth, or indeed any reassurance at all.

I remember what it can do beyond feeling pain. When dressing, there is a freedom to pause that hasn't been there for many months of colder weather. I let my bare limbs feel the warm air. I look at the soft curves of my hips and stomach in the mirror, and I wonder.

I run a bath and lie in it, watching the steam rise from my skin, and I think about desire. I let the pulse of its knowing find its way around my body, testing, pulling myself under the water to stop myself from shivering. A single air bubble loosens from the seaweed of my hair and bobs a line slowly down between my shoulder blades. The fuchsia seedlings on the windowsill shake in the breeze of the open window. I listen to the call of gulls and think about their pink mouths.

Desire is something women are supposed to facilitate in another, not feel in self-assured isolation. We are not supposed to keep it to ourselves. We are expected to inspire and inspire well, inspire beautifully and enticingly, and so my unshaved, aching legs prickling in the cold air, the faded knickers crumpled on the laminate, feel like both a transgression and a victory. This moment is not an invitation to anyone, and I can feel it, feel my full and singular ownership of it, here in this flawed, painful body.

In the early morning, there comes that warm pull again. To touch and forget, to ride the wave of something outside of myself, to make my body do something good, something just for me. I am amazed how often I don't think of doing it and the inevitability of it when I do, like remembering to take deep breaths.

I touch, then, and I try to find the right picture to accompany the act: the right jigsaw fit to make my heart tighten and my fingers quicken. They rise like pages turning – old lovers' hands, faces – but they are all lost and past, unreachable. I cannot pull them to me.

It is a grey sky I fix on in the end, to my surprise. Head back in damp grass, the lines of upside-down pylons stretching their power away from me, and the sound of geese, urgent and foreign, over my head, filling the sky. A language for us and for no one else; their personal, necessary cry my own; the clouds my full and ancient need. I come to the dark, wet grass and the wingbeat, and the strength of the imaginary, open steel above me, tall and mine.

Maybe desire can mean deep earth as much as it can quick hands? Maybe I belong to the sky as much as I do to anyone else now. Maybe I have grown that big, that connected, and, if I'm honest with myself, that overlooked. There is certainly more room for pain here.

How little time any desire gets to grow in, though; to answer itself or decide what it wants. I should get up. I should get on. My son needs his breakfast and ah, guilt: there you are. I wonder if my desire will ever get to exist without it.

I already think I should leave these words out. But then, how else to be my whole self?

★

THEN

I remember laughing again. I remember a lightness and energy in me, just sometimes. I found that I could draw it up and in from colour and life around me. It had been a long time since I'd been able to do that.

Some days, from my ever-quivering place, there could be an opening now, a flare. I could push through the overwhelming urge that seemed to pour from everything to speak, to leap, to grin. I realised I could be bold and clever, funny, surprising. I could make people laugh. I could make them feel good. These sudden sparks made people stop and notice me. It made boys like me. Even the boy I had longed for and who seemed to hate me for reasons I could never understand, even he noticed, his head turning, his smile softening just a little; one kiss, just one. It made girls jealous. Jealous of *me*!

I relearnt a quiet, vibrant intensity. I held my head a little higher. I brushed mascara onto my eyelashes to make them black, black; painted smoky grey around my eyes. I saw how it could make good things happen.

Then there were the days that I couldn't; when all I could do was curl and retreat, balled up tight again as I listened to people talk and laugh around me, trapped behind the tables of bars, trapped in my head, a silent scream, wanting to get out, get *out*. Like dough pulled apart and pushed back together again, I opened and closed, dived in, recoiled. I bounced from freedom and joy to confusion and frustration.

There came a question that I would ask and ask: how could I have this much light and courage in me and yet feel so overcome?

★

I put my headphones on. It is a practised movement.

It is hard to stay inside just now. Always that itch, that pull. I wish I could trust it and follow it wherever it wants to take me, but I know I can't. I don't want to lose too much time to inevitable recovery. I want time to watch the world and see what it has to show me. I want to find better ways of being out in it because I love it so, even though it drains me dry. I want to *live*. Isn't it obvious? I am not made to stay at home all the time.

The solution must simply be a matter of continued adaptation, I'm sure of it. I am trying to embrace that. Today that means a busier coffee shop than I'm used to, but armed, ready. Mum has parked me up in my wheelchair with my notebook and fetched a drink. She'll be back in an hour or so.

My sensitivity to sound has the lyrical name of hyperacusis and is severe enough now to demand noise-cancelling headphones. Wearing them is the difference between being able to last ten minutes outside or an hour. It isn't simple noise itself I struggle with as much as its overlap. Music over chatter over coffee-machine roar and hand-dryer hum leaves me crumpled, my body a banshee wail. I hear everything, every single thing, and I wilt under its intensity. If I muffle it all or give myself just one sound or one voice to listen to, I do better, my body releasing like a flicked switch, and so I seek that out, when I can. Piano music works best. Something gentle and rhythmic.

I am discovering that it comes with an odd side effect: I love people more when I can't hear them. Block my ears and I am suddenly, infinitely fuller of all the things I wish I was the rest of the time – love, compassion, patience. Muffle the world and I am abundantly adoring of one and all. I don't know why. Perhaps it's because it lets me notice things.

Without sound, I find that I watch people's hands. I notice who puts them to their mouths or their hair, who reaches for something to fill them, who interlaces them neatly. Without sound, I find I read eyes and watch lips. I see whose move most. There is a scale of softness to both lips and eyes and I like spotting the spectrum of them, looking at the faces on which they live. There are eyes that laugh even when their owners' faces are still; those that look around them, receptive or wary; more that hold a subtle hardness.

Freckles and moles are a special delight: those personal constellations. So are the ways people touch each other and themselves, distractedly, impulsively. I like to see how people fit together, how certain hands and arms reach to find each other in sudden, unspoken agreement. I love people's hair, especially when strands escape containment to fall over foreheads or be tucked behind ears. I love the way foreheads change like clouds change.

I like to see the space people take up and the way they shift around in it; the movements you know are habitual and practised and those that are not. I like to see where people's gazes and bodies rest, if they ever do; the ways they navigate others around them and whether they look at them directly, notice them, or wander an isolated corridor all their own. I love belly swells, the soft places and lines that shape each person and change each shadow.

I like to read mood and watch it alter, to suddenly see someone's teeth when before there was only a restrained, closed line. Openness in a face is rare, obvious warmth glowing only from the occasional one, and you see how people are drawn to that, like sunbathers. Most people have a turned-in quality, a watchfulness, but that is its own tender beauty and I love that too. You can tell who's listening and who isn't, and you can spot humour the easiest of all. It flickers in people a room away.

Then there are things that stand out – the oddities. A carefully curled moustache, looming height, a particularly graceful glide. They are easy to find: all you do is half close your eyes and wait for the thing that wakes you to attention. The tilt of the girl with heart-shaped mirror shades who has melted to the shape of her father's shoulder, bright wellies dangling. Identical twins, same coats, same expressions. The man with two missing front teeth.

My ears are starting to burn. I take my headphones off and there, ah the shame of it, I am lost to it all again, my own defences and story soon too thick to see through, my own thoughts and pain too loud.

All I want is to go home and be away from everyone.

★

THEN

It is May. I am running. Running down a dirt track under birch trees, the light racing with me and I am laughing. We were late, late. Too long spent doing things we shouldn't in the wood. I didn't care. I didn't care about anything that day, but no, I must slow down. There was more that happened first.

I was sixteen. My parents had announced that they were 'having problems'. The news landed in me without surprise, as a knowledge I had learnt before and forgotten. I said I was fine, that I knew everything would be fine, and avoided looking at my brother.

Very little changed. Mum and Dad simply moved around each other and around us, occupying different spaces in the practised way we had long lived. It drew no attention to itself, except for those times when I would hear muffled words from the utility room where we kept the washing machine. I'd stand there for a moment, wondering if I had walked into the closed door in front of me after all, my whole body vibrating with the impact. I'd walk away before I could think too much about it, too afraid to put my ear to it.

My parents were unravelling, but I had a new boyfriend now and my boyfriend's mum and dad were not unravelling. They were rock solid. I fell in love with them, with their not-divorcing, with their unbroken unit.

My new boyfriend's dad was tall and gentle and talked to me about cameras and photography. His mother was round and soft and clucked like a hen and made you feel like you knew exactly where you were. I remember her bare arms and the creases of his lined face. I remember the smell of their dog; the white teeth of his clowning little sister. My boyfriend himself was cool and funny. He dyed his hair so blond it went green.

Time at their house with all of them was some of the happiest I had known for years. I leaned into the warmth of it, not really caring that this boy drew only vague affection from me and no deeper feeling. This was safe. I liked this. I could make all these people feel good, easy as anything. My boyfriend seemed a little ashamed of me in public, but that was OK, I was a little ashamed of me too, and he was nice to me in the quiet of their house with its boxy rooms. It felt like home.

I had made a new friend by then too. I loved my other friends at the time, but always felt afraid with them. I never told them that. This one, though, she made me feel like I might be OK: Amelie.

I am more aware of my solitude again these last few weeks. I know why but I cannot speak the reason aloud yet; I'm not ready. Suddenly, there is too much space – there is all this *room* around me. I find myself wishing for it to be filled, like a belly is filled.

It is making me newly aware of my skin and how little connects with it. It is hard not to feel cold and small in this feeling of vastness. I get lost in it. It makes me want to collide with something bigger than me, something with pulse and vitality. I want to touch life, and have it touch me back. To feel all joined up, somehow. I want to be *needed*. Oh, the curse of all this spring sunshine.

I drift. I sigh. I open the back door. And the garden welcomes me with patient, open arms. I step into them once again.

There, I find it: that joining. My hands have work to do, and here there is a receiving of my labour, an acquiescence, a yielding that makes me feel whole, solid, seen. I sit again on the dirty floor, abandon gloves and trowels, and push into the sticky compost like a midwife. I tip seeds, sleeping, into my cupped palm and paw through them, selecting life, selecting futures, and the seeds do nothing but wait and trust.

There is such tender intimacy in it, such nurturing. I attend to each thing with a careful, deliberate confidence.

I look up and notice that the white clematis has grown into a tight knot, clutching desperately at itself with dry, hard tendrils. I go over and trace the stems of it, running my hands along its lines from the soil up to its highest shoots, under, over, through its tangle, seeing where to snip carefully, to draw individual vines apart. Under my gaze, it gradually starts to open, to open and loosen, until all its new growth can be spread wide and tied to supports in expansive submission. It can breathe now, I can feel it, and I feel worth course through me in response that I could minister to it.

I tease crowded seedlings apart too, pushing a finger into the soil to make a new, hollow nest for them in their own pots, tucking their filaments down with sure hands. I imagine them feeling safe. The bleeding heart holds up crystal balls of rainwater for me to peer into and bless. The rose trusts me with my secateurs to take what is needed from its over-eager shoots, to coax its shape from it. Things I thought dead push new heads above the soil and I know their name. When the apple tree finally blossoms soon, I know that there will be seven flowers in each cluster, although each is still clenched tight for now. What an honour it is to hold the memory of something when it has forgotten itself.

Here, I can be myself. The garden welcomes my keen hands and my broken feet. I sit with it and soothe and tend and it does nothing in response but grow. It pours itself into the space around me until there are no gaps left to feel. I can't be too much here. I can only be just right. It is such a perfect alignment of love and need that I hardly dare blink.

Listen. A wren is singing. A driver is leaning on his horn. A spider like a breadcrumb has fallen from my hat onto its back. In three good kicks it has turned to scuttle down the highway of my lined page as I write these words. I think its twin might be working its way down between my shoulder blades. Today, I think I might be brave enough to take some risks and start all over again. To leap off a hat and to test the edges of myself with nothing but belief in my own resilience and a long, deep breath.

★

THEN

Unlike the rest of us, Amelie appeared fully formed. She wore smudges of glitter-gel on her eyelids and cut up her clothes to patch them back together again in new ways: a freedom I could barely comprehend. When she twisted her blonde hair into knots and clips, they stayed there. Amelie's mum was an art teacher and her dad something important, I forget what. They were all impossibly beautiful, exuding bohemia. Her mother would push great curtains of hair back from her face while laughing, sexy in a way no other mums I knew were. She invited me to call her by her first name, but I never could bring myself to do it.

Their house was set high up on the hill in the best part of town, two minutes from my high school. It was the kind of house with a deep, balding scatter of loose stone before the bay window that crunched in an expensive way. We were preparing for our exams and in our free revision periods, we'd sneak up there and let ourselves in with her key. We'd wrap ourselves in duvets and watch American TV shows I'd never seen before on their satellite television and make beautiful GCSE revision cards. It didn't matter if you felt tired there. Comfort and rest became our play. Light poured through the wide windows onto the shelves and shelves of books that filled the rooms. The long kitchen held a tall refrigerator. The relative wealth of my friends was always revealed most starkly by the refrigerator. If it stood alone and was rounded rather than detention-block square, if it had a large, cold handle rather than a grubby notch in the door, then your friends were doing better than you – or their mum and dad were in comparison to yours, at least. It was the same thing back then.

And you'd think for all of this, for the back garden you couldn't see all in one glance and the moulded fireplaces and the sewn-on patches on her GAP coat, you'd think I would have resented her, but I didn't. I worshipped her. There was an ease to her and not a scrap of meanness. She had the kind of confidence of spirit that comes when you grow up being certain that there will always be more for you, so it doesn't matter if someone else takes some.

I loved her for her humour, her surety, and the way she made fun feel gentle and easy. I loved her for what she made feel possible. I loved her because she liked me, and because I knew I could make her feel wanted too.

One day, an eclipse fell. I don't remember when in my story it happened, but no one else was home so we climbed out of her bedroom window onto the extension roof and tried not to look at it. We huddled together, bare arms touching, our eyes down. I remember the light fading around me, the sudden, eerie finality of the birds, the goosebumps on my skin, the paleness of hers, both saying nothing at all, not needing to say anything at all, not needing to be anything but right there.

There is joy in the moments when you and those around you slot into life like its missing pieces, like you were everything it had been looking for, and you know yourself perfect, just for a moment. I felt transcendent, happier and simpler than I'd ever been. No games to play. Nothing to figure out. Nothing to do but watch the slow shift of it, as the day woke up again from its artificial dark.

I was getting better then, I think. I was healing. If only I'd had more time, but I was invited to go on holiday with my boyfriend's family – the five of us and the dog – to a caravan on the Welsh coast. 'You can go, as long as you revise.' That was the deal, and I nodded my usual yes yes yes.

And I did revise, a little, but mostly I let my legs catch the late spring sunshine and catch my boyfriend, and rode bikes and rode him too, and I didn't care, I didn't care, because I was running, and I was away from home, and I was free, and that's when it happened.

I tripped on a root and hit the ground hard. I was up again, laughing within seconds, but by the time I got home the pain was extraordinary. I couldn't speak. I couldn't move. I was half-carried from their old Land Rover and delivered into the hands of my white-faced parents.

I remember a long night upright, moaning and rocking in the dark, a doctor injecting me with something sharp and cold.

Hospital lights. Surgery on my hip. Three more weeks in hospital and a long, long recovery. My GCSE exam dates passed by one by one. English, Science, Maths, History, Art. All of them. All missed. All lost.

I tumbled, and I didn't stop.

★

I reach for my phone, read the text, and freeze.

I feel it come: the fall, the jolt. Something rips. I feel myself wake up in this new place with no oxygen in it and try to take a breath and feel my lungs open and close, empty. It is just for a moment, before the world shifts again, and I look down at my feet and see that I am still here somehow, still breathing somehow, calm under the sunshine, a new ache in my chest.

A friend of mine has died. He was so young. He's had cancer for a long time, and I love him. Loved him.

I say, 'God, no.' Time spins. For a long while, I don't think at all, and then I think, 'I know this feeling', and I am not alone in my day any more.

The older you get, the harder it is to experience a singular grief. Instead, when loss comes again, it doesn't bring something solid all the way through or isolated, it brings you a Russian doll. Loss comes; a new layer of grief forms. And instead of staying still, it *opens,* and out all the others pour, popping into their composite forms until you are sitting surrounded by an eager, bleeding crowd of them. Grief is cumulative and to feel one kind is to feel at least a little of them all, renewed. When I wake from the shock, there it is, right here in my hands. All my past losses, nestled.

I sit in the garden and remember my friend and try to let all my dolls emerge from this new grief. I try not to fight it or to be afraid, to let them unpack through all my past losses and trauma, right down to the smallest parts of myself. They just want to be close to this thing they know, close to my friend and this splintering shift in the world, that's all. They mean no harm.

I try to sit with all of them in peace, held together by this new layer that isn't mine to claim as my property but which I feel a piece of all the same because I loved him, and I love the people who loved him, and because it isn't fucking fair. And I weep for a long time, in the high, safe walls where no one can see me and that is right and good.

Grief makes me feel more connected to other people than almost anything else. There is no single emotion we get to claim as solely our own, but I think grief may be the most shared, the most universal. I would hope love too, but that seems to be more fragile somehow, less guaranteed. There is grief in that too.

I am always so aware that each of us takes turns at this, handing it around like hot boulders. It has always struck me that though we talk of loss, grief feels like an addition. Something is taken from you, but at the time, it feels like something is added. Something weighty and burning and wide. Here, this is yours now, it says.

There is a peaceable balance to it, in a way: a companionship. So much in life is lonely, but grief doesn't need to be. You cannot experience it alone entirely – what you feel is shared by multitudes – and I find comfort in that. In my adult, ageing body, it feels newly right to make space for grief as part of daily life. It feels like a way to honour my humanity, my mortality, and the humanity and mortality of those around me. I know I live more deeply and more lovingly for the appreciation of it.

As I grow, I can recognise its shape more and more in the people I meet. It's like seeing something hand-shaped. I will always think 'hand' to myself if I see that shape, knowing that it is linked to my own. I can press mine to it and though its size and form may differ, I will still feel a sense of fit, a recognition. I think grief works the same way. I see yours and though it is not mine, I know something of it, enough of it that I can be with you in its experience, and that is something miraculous.

It is so simple, really, and yet also not at all. Something is gone, suddenly, devastatingly, and we fall into the gap it leaves. Our universe's laws are broken, unreality no longer unreal, while all around us the world seems just the same, as if it didn't know a part of itself had been pulled inexorably apart. How could we stay unchanged through that? How could we not be undone? When time itself becomes hard to grasp. When tenses knock against our teeth. He is? He was? That there should suddenly be a before and after. That we have always lived, drawing towards this moment without knowing. Was I? Will I be? I know it, but I do not understand it. I expect I never will. It is in all this we huddle together, each with our weights, our Russian dolls.

This is the beauty and the muddle and pain of grief, and humility cuts through it like a migraine because underneath it all, I know I still don't know grief as well as I will do, one day. All lives lead inevitably, cumulatively, to that deeper knowing.

For now, I stand. I water my sunflowers. I touch careful hands to those I love; to those I wish to love more.

There is nothing else to do.

★

THEN

I don't remember. I don't remember. It's all mixed up, and I can't get it to make sense. I am in the car sobbing over a piece of paper that says F F F F all the way down. I am being wheeled to the toilet, showering in a cold plastic chair. I am kneeling on a hard floor, resolutely cheerful and smiling as always, measuring socked feet in a shoe shop, my name on my chest. I am saying goodbye and goodbye and goodbye. To hold it together makes my head hurt. Can all of this have been me?

There are simple things I know to be true. I returned to school in the autumn, my hip healing, but with a new sensation like a soft thrum of sound from my waist down. They could find no reason for me to be in so much pain still – the injury and resulting infection had been severe, but they could see no lasting damage. New pain joined old until it all settled into something like background noise. I tried to pick up the threads of my life again.

It was decided I would re-sit some of my missed GCSEs alongside studying for A levels and I attended double classes to try and catch up. My dad moved out and leaned on me, frightened, lost. My green-haired boyfriend dumped me, or I dumped him. I don't suppose it matters. Some days, I wasn't sure whose parents I missed. His or my own? Some days, I wondered if I missed something else entirely. Something I had lost, or never had at all.

★

The women sit on the grass on the horizon and their three shapes make a skyline. I lie a little way down the slope, failing to read my book in the sun.

May is getting warm now; warm enough to throw off unnecessary clothes. The women's voices are gravelly with nicotine, their thin hair scraped back into low ponytails. They wear vest tops and tracksuit bottoms in black and grey, with one, lone football shirt making a blazing red tulip in the grass.

They hold lager cans in one hand, cigarettes in the other. Their shoulders are thin and hunched, defensive, their words loud. They talk of their evictions, their probation officers, of Tommy and Mick and Gav, and play out long, complex confrontations in a torrent of 'he said' and 'I said'. The words come and go with the wind, the odd, raised, 'I fucking told him' carrying like plastic flotsam on the tide.

I am happy to be here with them at first, nearby and nodding in the dandelions over my remembered picnic blanket. I am glad they are enjoying the sunshine – glad we all are. They are my neighbours and this is our home. I have walked a whole fifteen steps here from my mobility scooter, left beside the footpath, calculated to leave it behind me but not so far that I'll be marooned after an hour of sitting. They looked, of course – people always look – but haven't looked a second time. Apart from another woman asleep on her back nearer the lake, we are alone.

Their pale skin is mottled. They all look like broken glass, like abandoned industrial lots, and I worry for them and wonder for them, how is it the three of them had met, bunched around these cauldrons of their fraught and complicated lives. They are maybe forty, forty-five, or look it, at least. I can know from a dozen metres away that their lives have been hard and cruel, with unkindness received and inevitably cascading from them in turn at times, because how could it not? When it's pressed into you enough, that's often what leaks from your edges. And even knowing this, I begin to stiffen with it, lying there, so much spite and harshness pouring from them.

They are a skyline more and more, all sharp corners and unlit places, all torn-up pavement, all dug-up roads. The chaos of them is like a traffic roar. It is overwhelming, especially here in this place of shifting grass and blue sky and gentler birdsong than their own.

Engine noise, for real now. We all turn, for we are at the far edge of a stretch of land that holds the graveyard in its middle and there is no road nearby. A car is driving over the mown verge, around the graves and the trees, over the grass that borders them. It turns in a wide circle, flattening daisies, revving its engine and filling the air with fumes, and the women stand and whoop and laugh and smack their knees as it stops beside them. A sticker in the back window proclaims *TOP HUNTER* and I shiver.

A reedy, pinched man gets out and bows to his prizes as they too bend double with the glee of it. He hands over a packet of something. I do not know if he is Tommy or Mick or Gav, but he adds his own chaos for a while and then leaves with another wheel-spinning circle on the grass, to thread his way back through the dead to the distant road, leaving the women to laugh again and declare what a legend he is, what a solid bloke, and I wonder, I wonder.

Soon, two more men have joined them, the kind whose smiles don't reach their eyes and whose fists are all gristle. The woman no longer asleep by the lake rouses and leaves, face hard.

That hardness has formed inside me too. I feel
the instinctive shutter-down of it. There has been a
turning away in me, a distancing – like cutting a rope
and watching something drop. I think about leaving
too, but the beauty of this place, so rarely visited,
makes me hold my seat. 'I'll leave if there's trouble,'
I think, and those fifteen steps to my scooter feel like
too many.

But there is none. The only one with spikes bared is
me as I sit, rigid and unfocused. They lie at ease with
each other and the day until, like geese in the fields
shifting towards flight, they all stand at once to leave.

The wind drops and the final exchange of them
arrives like another quiet package pressed into my
own hands.

'Have you got all your rubbish? I'm not having you
fucking littering.' It is the tallest woman, hair like a faded
rabbit-hutch, straps loose against thin shoulders. 'I tell
you, I hate it. It fucks me right off when people do that.'

The others laugh, uncomfortable and look away,
but she continues, unabashed, gathering the detritus of
them all into the carrier bag they brought the beer in.

'When I was a kid, in Bristol,' she says, 'we lived
by this common, right, all grass and stuff, and one
Saturday me and me sister, we robbed some bin bags
and picked up all the litter. Took all day, it did. I'll
never forget it.'

The others are helping too now, half-heartedly, and I watch them, my complicated wombles, their quieter words lost from me again until they slouch to the path without another look.

I think I make a noise like a sob, but it is lost in the wind and the grass and the blackbird in the hedgerow.

How much I still have to learn, about prejudice, and tenderness, about faithfulness and the secret goodness of people; where it's found and how to stay open to it. How not to miss it.

★

THEN

Life expanded and retreated at a dizzying rate. I recall it like a great heave of bellows, a juddering oscillation. All is out of sync. Memories of happiness flare like lit matches, bright and then spent.

I remember a new Saturday job in a clothes shop and the rattle of the hangers, the colour of the garments, the colours of each textbook I pored over in the evenings, a sting in my eyes, the endless lamplight. I remember confusion and the overwhelming terror of subtext, how everyone and everything swam with it. I knew what people said didn't match their eyes, but I couldn't understand it: this constant, low-level unease.

I remember laughing until I cried; Amelie in winter sunshine, wrapped in bright scarves. I remember running away to a dirty city with a man in his twenties for a night and my drink being spiked and not knowing what I did next. I remember sitting in the garden at home and watching a spider build a web, point by point as the evening got darker and darker, refusing to come in, wondering if I could just stop there and be done with it all. I remember a desperate, mindless promiscuity.

I remained outwardly quite calm in the middle of it all. I was always affable, always compliant. I kept so much hidden because I had no idea what I was doing or what to say. I was delightful. I was thoughtless and unkind. I was unbelievably stupid. I was always so much at once.

★

I don't know what to do today so I will make a cup of tea. There is nothing else for it. I have forgotten everything. I have no idea what the hell anything means or who I am supposed to be or what I'm supposed to be doing. I am all blank, all gone, but for this one thread of me left. Look, it leads to the kitchen. I will follow it until I reach the kettle and then I will make a cup of tea and everything will be OK again, maybe. Maybe it will.

How funny that drinking tea is the one act of hope that endures; the one thing that resists falling through that trapdoor of panic and despair. You could lose faith in everything else, but you would still take a cup of tea held out, I know you would. On the days when I can barely stand my face in the mirror, I will still, carefully, kindly, brew myself a cup of the stuff. It is an untouchable parlay. A gap in the wall. A truce in the most complicated feeling of everything.

It is history too. Every cup is full of the others. The repetition of it allows all of me to be in one place at the same time, just for a little while, rather than pulled apart and scattered like I usually am. Hold a cup and I am back together, joined by cups of tea past. What a relief to be whole. No wonder I make so many.

I sip, and my legs are strong again and pushed back through the long, damp grass under a hedgerow. I have been walking. The reflection of hawthorn berries and field maple and sky make the black, still surface of the water look like I've filled the thermos cup full of everything I could find around me.

A different cup, another sip away, rests on my knees as I sit in the dirt of the back doorstep watching the streetlamp pulse on, listening to the blackbird sing sweet jazz to the bins in the ginnel.

Another sip and I am holding the scrunched slumber of my new-born son against my shoulder, pawing nervously with my other hand to try and reach the mug gone cold that is over there, somewhere.

They are all in there.

Every cup brewed after a bad night, after shock, after pain, the trauma only making it taste all the better – oh, it is a dark magic, that. Every day that felt like it would never end. Every first time asked, shyly, 'How do you take it?' Every long, naked back watched possessively and languidly, swinging its way out of bed to dutifully fetch it just the way I like it. Every one made for no one but myself, defiant, lazy, distracted, brave, with no witnesses at all.

We are all made witches in its brewing. We mutter words over its surface, shaky hands stirring, hoping it might help the next moment go our way. I have made some mugs with love so feverish and potent, the water could boil again through sheer will; others with a crack and clench and hiss of ice. Each has been a spell, intention and feeling heaped in. Some designed, if only secretly, to meld, hold, bind. Others to construct a careful barrier of propriety and protection.

I can list half a dozen people I secretly wish to make tea for, to mark a first cup with. Another dozen where every new cup would feel like a victory against change, against ending and death; a jubilant, resounding 'HA!' because I'd have got to have made you another, and that would mean we'd beaten it all for a little while longer. And then there are the shadowy few where the longing to make them just one more, just *one*, is so fierce and enduring that I have to stop myself reaching for an extra mug, and sometimes I do, I'll admit, leaving it cold on the counter.

For now, I hold this cup alone, this very latest one in the chain. I hold it in aching hands and smile. I know who I am. Tea-witch, lover, mother, daughter, friend.

★

THEN

I will tell you what I know.

Before long, something in me burnt out. I dropped out of high school and everyone was horrified – me most of all. I spent the summer regrouping and avoided going home, sleeping at friends' houses as often as I could. In the autumn, I smiled my way into an assistant manager position at a small, sleepy shoe shop which I enjoyed every day. I loved knowing exactly what was expected of me, the smell of the leather, the neat boxes in the stockroom. I took part-time classes at the local college to try and reclaim some A levels while I worked, and for a while, everything seemed OK again.

I turned eighteen and met the man I would marry, grinning at him shyly over the CD racks in the music shop he worked in, enamoured by his blue eyes, his eyebrow ring. Together, we watched my dad walk down the aisle with a woman I had barely begun to know, my role as his emotional support suddenly, startlingly no longer needed.

I watched my friends leave town and go to university, my blonde-haired, laughing Amelie too. I only saw her one more time after that, awkward, changed, and the fresh loss settled inside me like new bones.

And my mother told me, shaking with an alien terror, that she was gay and in love with her best friend. She waited for judgement, for to me to hate her. I held her instead, crying with her saying, 'I knew, I knew', because I did, and I felt more love in that moment than I'd ever felt before, all rifts healed.

I know I got sicker and sicker and slower and slower.

I tried to keep going – I did. I tried not to indulge this body that they told me would only get worse with more attention, but I was so tired, so tired all the time.

★

It has been another hard day. It is still painful to admit how many I have. I had plans to work, to move, to be brave, but I have done nothing but sit hunched, pain loud, thoughts louder, a frightened child again. The day has cycled past my window and now it's gone. I sit in the dark, resisting sleep, staring at the half-empty glass on my bedside table, stagnant with yesterday's water. I don't want to accept that I've lost another twenty-four hours. I don't want to be this. Not again.

I do believe very deeply in loving the body you're in. How could I not? Without its help, little else can continue. You learn that fast and sharp when you get sick or are badly hurt, and then you forget it just as quickly. When you've been ill a long time, you forget it in a different way. You tune out your body or write it off as a lost cause. You see it as trash you must inhabit, little more than that. A cage, a shackle. You can do the same to your mind. I have done this. I do this.

The veins on my hands are beginning to form raised ridges; the knuckles of my long fingers beginning to collect finer and finer lines. I look at them in the light of the lamp that I do not want to switch off. They look just as my mother's hands did when I was small. I knew of no greater comfort then.

The day's last minutes tick past and I think: I don't want to spend my life trapped in something I hate and resent. That is a dark life and my days are restricted enough. I want to show my body, my mind, that it still matters to me, that I believe it is good. If I don't, if I do nothing but fill it with hate and fear every day, I know I will lose the last and most precious, enduring relationship of my life. I know I will poison it and the trust between us and then I really will be alone because nothing else can take its place. Besides, even if I did hate it, hate myself, it wouldn't change a damn thing. I know because I've tried that. This way is better.

Put something fragile, vulnerable and newly alive in my arms and the world would see me care for it with an attention and good humour that could change the world. I would be so gentle: sweet voice, careful, loving touch. I would be the mother my son knows. The mother I remember. And yet this tangle of muscle and bone, this pumping heart, these busy thoughts: these are what have got me this far. *This* is the form that will see me through all the rest of my days, whatever shape it's in, whatever it looks like, however much it struggles. These are the only hands that will let me stroke and soothe the people I love, the only back that will root me when I need to hold firm. My breath is the only space that will allow me to pause and gather myself in and maybe finally, finally do what's right. My mind is the only one I get to work with. This is my one ride.

So many of us search endlessly for some sense of a lasting home and forget that we already inhabit it. However imperfect, our body is the one thing that's ever really ours. It's the one thing we get to keep hold of all our life.

It is hard though. It is so hard, I know. I am struggling to hold true to these things today; my body full of rage, my mind full of panic. That is why I write this: to choose love, to remember.

I try a new thing. I reach out to the wolf. It is all snap and bite in this bed, but I know that is because it is afraid. I don't want it to be afraid.

I place shaking fingers against the skin of my own arm. I stroke, soft, soft. Shh. Be still. It's OK. It's OK.

I cry. Of course I do.

★

THEN

It was like before: the complete incapacity of my younger days. The dragging fatigue, the stripped-wire pain. I got myself to two college exam re-sits and let the third go as a lost cause. No one intervened. I had missed months of lectures – the lecturers barely knew my name. My hours at the shoe shop dwindled until I had to quit. I could barely stand, and there was no 'next', no friends, no mentors, no prospects, no plan, so for now I simply went home from my last exam and lay down.

My mother saved up and paid for me to visit a private doctor as a one-off. He looked at my notes, at the years of unexplained symptoms, and spoke past me to tell her, briskly, that this was a picture of mental imbalance, not physical. It was best not to indulge me with fantasies of disease again. He prescribed exercise and activity and to focus on something other than myself. He took her money while I stared out of the window at the rolling green expanse of his garden.

Mum frowned behind the wheel all the way home, furious, her gear changes jerked and aggressive, while

I looked straight ahead and tried to apologise. She was adamant that it was lazy, assumptive rubbish, but I believed him, still, back then.

I wasn't a child any more, threatened by some idea of a dangerous sadness. I felt no real stigma about mental health issues, only a kind of academic interest. I had taken Psychology as an A level subject, fascinated by the interplay of mind and experience. I knew that there was a link between body and thought; behavioural and neurological traps that your brain could fall into without realising it. I didn't feel particularly anxious but there was no escaping the fact that my mind was complex and that it had suffered. Perhaps it was to blame after all. Perhaps it always had been, in ways I couldn't comprehend, although I didn't understand why that made me immune to sympathy or support. I didn't want to ignore the possibility. I wanted to look directly at it. I wanted to fix it.

I lay for a long time in the bed with the white sails still draped over it and thought about what to do to tame this error inside me. I looked at my mind. I turned it over and over for weeks on end, but all I could find was confusion, hope and determination: always, that roaring desire to live. It was immensely frustrating. How could I fix this if I didn't have anything to work with?

This was supposed to be the time all young birds flew, and I had not flown, could not. I wanted to understand. How unkind it had been for the adults in my life to spend my whole early life telling me how much potential I had, how I would go far if I tried – to university and on to a shining career. It had set a level of expectation, of assurance: it had promised me that's how life worked. It made all deviations feel like failure because they had told me success only looked like one thing. School never taught me about change, chaos, fluidity, adaptation, and so I knew nothing of those things. All I knew was that I'd broken some pact by failing to conform and now no one wanted to help me.

I would be good now, I'd tell myself, I pleaded with the air; I had learned my lesson. I don't know who I said these things to, what lesson I was supposed to have learnt. I guess the concept of God dies hard.

My little brother was at college too now and I would wake from long sleep to the sound of his key in the door. We'd boil the kettle and talk about his day. He had grown tall, intense, his eyes dark, his hair thick and adamant, and with little left to distract me, I saw him and loved him in a new way – as equals, as teammates. I loved him, and loved my mother's blossoming under the care of the woman she loved and who loved her back, and I loved my dad with a confused ache too, as he began a new, more distant life with new, younger step-children and a wife with a sharp tongue.

★

I am looking at the grape hyacinths nodding over my notebook. I am looking at my bare legs, the raised hairs on my arms, the gleam of my hands in the bright sun. Something has happened to my breath lately. It is thicker. It flows in and out like something warm and liquid. I have to keep from swallowing over and over.

I do not know how to tell this. All these months writing boldly of a single life, of courage and solitude and self-sufficiency, and here this was waiting, as if to show me up.

I am falling in love. I feel like I must have got the tenses wrong, that I must be writing about the past again, but no, no, this is now. This is happening now. I am falling in love. I have already fallen. Oh, help.

They have started me on a new cardiac drug regime and it is working. Every time my nervous system tries to pull me into galloping tachycardia and unconsciousness at the slightest movement, the chemical pacemaker helps to steer me back. I am fainting less. There is a new safety and yet now I am not safe at all.

To have been pulled out of the symptoms of heart failure at the exact same time my heart was pulled so unexpectedly into new love is so ridiculous as to be unbelievable. I'm not even sure I trust it, believe in it, in sudden, determined love like this – love like a new magnetic north and your whole self pulled towards it. Do I? Do you? I feel like you will laugh at me. I wouldn't blame you for it.

I text him from my hospital bed, my heart rate already a steadier, more sensible line on the monitor just an hour after the drugs had hit my blood stream. I hoped it wouldn't jump when his answer came and ruin the whole procedure. I wondered if I should declare him.

'Are there any variables we should take into account?'

'Ah, yes, you see, there is this man . . .'

We pore over our early communications like mages over star maps, trying to understand it. How could simple sentences exchanged innocently as strangers have grown into this? A polite, formal correspondence, then shy and eager, shifting so quickly to avid, to unapologetically, joyously sure? This isn't the slow pace I am used to.

Eight weeks ago, he contacted me to thank me for some writing he'd read of mine and sent me money to buy spring plants with. 'No gardener should have to worry about their finances in springtime,' he wrote, and I felt the world sway. I returned with my surprise and thanks, and we began to write of our gardens, of poetry, and then of our souls, of course, hidden in both. Back and forth, the gaps between grew shorter and shorter.

Two months ago, I didn't even know his name and now it is a mantra, dug all the way into the soil of me. Fraser: his name is Fraser.

Words soon weren't enough. We've spent the last month hesitantly touching our fingers to the video screens that now sit between us every evening. He lives in another country, a beautiful one that he emigrated to over a decade ago. He shows me the sky there each day, a different blue to mine. He is fourteen years my senior – nearly fifty – but looks younger than his years, his hair thick and light brown, his jaw angular and strong. He takes his glasses off when he talks to me, worried they make him look too geeky, but I like them.

He has goodness running all the way through him. He has read every book I ever think to mention and can recommend five more, apologetically, without even trying. He looks down and his voice shakes when he says something vulnerable, but he speaks with an articulate honesty that makes my heart thump wild in my chest again. His wife left him, suddenly, last year.

I had thought I wasn't looking for love and yet to love him is now all I want to do. He had only meant to be kind, he had only hoped, maybe, to make a friend, and now I am all he can think of. 'What have you done to me?!' he laughs, his delighted fear palpable.

It is impossible and impractical, but we don't want to stop. I don't want to stop.

I have written of vulnerability so many times but how little I knew of it really until now. I know I have been wrong before. I know I have been blind. I know I have made devastating mistakes and thought I understood and didn't, but this, I think this is different, or could be. You must think me such a fool.

I have avoided writing about him these last few weeks, deliberately, stubbornly. I'm not even sure I should now. I am scared to break the spell. About the only thing I can bear to do is tend the garden, driven ever more desperately to try and make something grow. I poke sharp sticks into the soil around the newest, wobbliest additions and scatter toxic slug pellets with fierce understanding even though I'd sworn never to use them again. Don't touch my seedlings. Please.

The laughable, horrifying, beautiful alignment of it, to fall in love during springtime, when all around me fragile new things struggle towards a new life; a time when so many things fail. To still be in this body, this body I thought would never be enough for anyone again; to wonder and worry that all this is some horrible mistake and that something is waiting to devour it all as soon as I am assured. Life has done that so many times already, I cannot help but fear.

I have wept. I have lost all mindful composure. How hard it is to be present and clear seeing when everything in you reverberates with soon, if, but.

Suddenly, there is a 'next'. Suddenly, there are plans, dreams. It's as if life has nudged my whole, still earth back into movement. How much I underestimated the relentlessness of change. I have spent years in this house, this scattering of familiar streets, and now there is the potential of new sun on my shoulders. I am full of fire under this clear sky and a man I wonder if I could spend the second half of my life with shyly talks of all the things he wants to show me, to share with me.

I asked him if he would like to come away with me soon, to somewhere close and quiet, where we could get to know each other better. My son is going on holiday with his dad for a week and I thought, I could go somewhere too, couldn't I? And I could not go alone? He said yes, yes. It was the bravest thing I've ever done.

I do not understand how life can be this terrifying and this tender. I do not understand.

I am so happy. I am so very afraid.

★

THEN

My new boyfriend from the music shop stuck around. With all this love in me, it was easy to love him too. He was the best thing in my life and I kept close to his light. He was handsome and straightforward, undemanding and faithful. He worked hard and loved the things he loved – music, films – with a joy that was contagious. There was no dangerous passion in him or frightening desire. He hadn't broken or gone wrong or moved away or hurt me, and so I clung to him, determined to keep this one good thing as my own. We watched films together in his tiny box room on his single bed, every inch of wall and ceiling plastered over with posters. I said maybe we could live together one day. He nodded and smiled and said that sounded great and I felt the hope like an orchestra swell.

We talk of love as such a safe and spotless, unquestionable thing. We talk of beginnings that way too – as specific, pivotal moments, full of choice. A bold step. A clear *yes*. Sometimes they are. Sometimes, instead, beginnings are like looking up mid-thought and realising you are already moving. What else is there to do but sit back in your seat and continue? Sometimes it's the right way to go. Sometimes it isn't. The most terrifying thing of all is that, at first, it's impossible to tell.

★

Saturday morning. I sit on a chair, slowly knitting a cardigan, watching my son with his piano teacher. I try to keep the syncopating beat of my knitting needles quiet and unobtrusive. The window is open and the late May sun can't pretend any more: it is no longer the blushing girl of spring; it has grown hot and full and high.

My boy's feet don't quite touch the floor from the piano stool, not yet. He plays 'Ode to Joy' and I know I'll be humming it, absently, for the rest of the day. I do that when I'm noisy with overwhelming sensation – the same phrase over and over, compulsive, soothing – and I am overwhelmed today. I watch my son's nervous, hopeful face as he fumbles the notes for the dozenth time and looks for reassurance. His teacher responds with unabashed praise, with the subtlest of guidance, with pride. This morning sings with love. I think I am learning new things about that. When love is needed; when it makes the biggest difference to a life.

I sit and I knit. I cradle my new things: Fraser; hope; these tender stories I am writing down. I feel more vulnerable, more exposed, and more frightened than I think I ever have. It stops me, stills me, every few stitches. It fills my mouth, my throat. This joy is painful. It is a devastating desire. Some days, it's shaking me raw.

I know now what I must do. I know what all this is going to take. I must unclench, unfurl. I must shed my skin and become a new baby thing, ready to start again, terrible and bawling. I must turn, move my feet, and reach towards the things that suffering has told me *aren't meant for me*. Some days, I think about how much simpler it would be to stay in a hunched, dark place. How perversely comforting and affirming it would feel, to let the world confirm what I always feared: that I am no good anyway, that I only ever make mistakes, and so should save myself the time and upheaval and simply stay right here where it already hurts. There is pain in it, excruciating, but underneath, a safety, a logic. Suffering does make a sort of hollow sense, but I know the tragic lure of that. I know the snare. I watch it, wary.

We've both been doing it, Fraser and me. We've spent weeks trying to tell each other of all our worst flaws. I spell out how ill I get, as blunt and honest as I can manage. He says, 'I'm awkward and hopeless and nothing special.' Our phones ping with facts we've decided essential. 'I am averagely hairy, I think?' 'I couldn't walk today.' 'I thought you should know that I have good dental hygiene but weak, Scottish teeth.' 'I get very frightened.' 'My wife thought I was boring.' We apologise for everything we can think of. We drip feed our truths thinking that if the other turns away, at least it would be better for that to happen now.

Neither of us turns away. Still suffering, still bleeding, still secretly convinced of our unworth, we inch towards the other. We forget ourselves and talk for hours, about books, writing, philosophy, nature. He is clever, quick and full of energy. He makes me laugh and is delighted when he realises that he has. He sends me photographs from his long evening runs around the Danish countryside – that's where he lives. Lines of trees; neat, white churches; pictures of starscapes he's stayed up to take from cold beaches. He's a toymaker for the most famous toy company in the world. He hides and underplays his success until he can't, embarrassed by it. Our conversations carry through his trips to Canada, to Switzerland. He apologises again that his life is one of business meetings and conference calls, thinking I'll be repelled by it. He thinks my world far more interesting. I just want to know him, this quiet, exceptional man, whatever he says. I just want to brighten his days. I don't need anything else, please, just give me that.

There are moments of weighted silence filled with nothing but longing. We hold back from anything too ardent, but desire slips into our talk, testing, testing. Do you want me? Could you? we think, we hint. 'Some things are best saved for when we meet,' we say out loud.

I try not to break it. How easily I could. This is why we need love from the people around us when something starts to go well, or when it could. I tell you: our need for love doesn't stop when goodness finds us. If anything, it intensifies. We need to be loved more with each new time, each new chance, not less, for it is now, in these fragile first steps all over again, with the weight of our pasts on our shoulders, that we are most likely to panic. To decide we can't, we CAN'T. We don't deserve this. We're not good enough. We'll only fail again.

It is love's job to say, firmly: you can. You do. You are. You must try.

Jude and Mum ask me gentle questions. They make space for my new things. They let me talk, eager and embarrassed, frightened and fumbling, and I feel more love now than any kind word achieved in years of heartbreak and pain, because they believe I am worth this. They believe these new things are mine to have. I know that if these new seeds of mine get to grow into something strong and beautiful, it will be because I have been loved well through these shaky beginnings.

Perhaps all joy, all brave growth, and all bright achievement that exists in the world was built on love received like this once.

'One more time, from the beginning,' the piano teacher says.

We get nowhere alone. I think that's what I'm realising from this wonderful, terrifying place. We get nowhere alone.

Summer

We had said 'no expectations.' We had arranged for there to be a polite spare bedroom.

Now I can see his silhouette through the glass door of the holiday lodge before I open it. He looks small and far away. The last few feet are an impossible distance and I hope I don't faint. I might, and then what will we do? My mind is brave, but my body isn't. My body doesn't care about first impressions and I know it will crumple with no apology. I need it now. Please, please give me this.

I arrived yesterday, my mum dropping me at this place hidden in the Shropshire hills. She left me with my wheelchair, my suitcase, my nerve. I knew this was crazy: we all knew it was, but to be entirely dependent on other people to go anywhere at all is to have no secrets. My life now necessitates that I abandon all guile and become someone frank, someone who talks simply and says exactly what she means. I am glad of it. I have come to hate secrets. They are nothing but a collusion with yourself, a padding around truth when you're convinced that you need to protect something. Things fester in that dank, closed-off place and they eat it till it's spoiled. I wanted the windows open on this right from the start.

And so, I talked through this plan with Mum, Jude, even Dad. Fraser drew in his friends, confessing, red-faced. Together we worked out how I might make this leap safely, sanely – or at least as safe or sane as love and desire can ever be. Because I have been something fragile all my life, it can be hard for people to see beyond my vulnerability. They can end up wanting to keep me safe like a secret too, but the people in my life have all come to know my strength and my sense beyond appearances and they trust it. Mum and Jude had both said, 'Anything you need to make this happen, I'm here.' They had both hugged me tight and let me grin and blush at them like a new bride.

I slept alone last night in restless, dream-filled sprints, waking often. I tried to orientate myself to the small lodge that hangs over a bend in the river, finding the new handholds I need to get around. Help was only a call away if I needed it. I kept my phone close. 'Are you sure you still want me to come?' he asked, once, twice, and I replied each time, 'Yes. Yes, please come. It's beautiful here.'

The water runs unhurriedly under the balcony, under the trees. The damselflies are quick turquoise.

There is a wood burner and a row of well-worn paperbacks on the shelf beside it. It is warm, warm enough for bare feet and for me to have fallen asleep with the windows pushed wide while I waited for the sound of his rental car on the gravel. There were no sounds until then except the water, the whinny of horses behind the hedge on the far bank, a startled pheasant on the bridge.

I unlock and open the door and there he is. We say our shy hellos. He is shorter and thinner than I had thought, his face more lined, but soft, familiar. It is only then I realise that his first full sight of me will be my clumsy journey back to the sofa, unsteady and slow, but I try to hold my head high and act like it doesn't matter. He has made it clear that it doesn't matter.

We sit down, and for long moments I think all is lost after all; that he will fold in the middle, a crease from throat to stomach snapping him shut like a closed book. I don't think I have ever seen anyone look so exposed or so afraid, and to remember that, suddenly, that my vulnerability doesn't exist alone here, is to feel such relief that I have to stop myself from crying right in front of him. I am not the only one afraid. I try to breathe, chest tight. In his words, his gestures, his gentle, pleading eyes, I watch him hand all his power to me. He hands me a wounded, aged heart.

Eyes are one thing you can't see well through digital screens. His, I see only then, are tan and grey and green all at once. I talk to him in my simple, smiling way, and he talks back, and slowly we remember that we know each other. Slowly we realise that neither of us is disappointed.

It is him, in the end who reaches first – brave, brave – for my hand and then my waist as I lead him out to the balcony to show him the water. It is him who helps my head find his shoulder for just a moment of rest and reassurance. Each shared thing is a little key, a little breath.

The first cup of tea he makes for me is in a red mug with a chip in it. He has talked for weeks of how he'd like to make me tea and so hands this first one to me sincerely, like an offering. He hasn't noticed the chip and, as I drink, I smile again and press my lip to the curve of the powdery hollow – softly. There is a pulse in me. We begin to talk of how we might care for each other, how we both want to. We begin to draw closer and closer. He apologises for the chip. I say it is perfect.

The next morning, he brings me another mug, unchipped, with two round biscuits on a plate. I sit up in our new, shared bed and eat them carefully with both hands, thoughtful, still waking from the surprise of our first night together, the crumbs falling around me. He laughs at me, charmed, his head to one side, his bare torso already familiar, the curve of his ribs sweeping wide to his breastbone like a ship's prow. I have never felt so safe. I wonder how that could be.

Was I always afraid before? Can something as big as fear hide in plain sight? I think it can. I think it hides behind the secrets we keep from each other – those aspects of ourselves we're too terrified to show. I feel this safe because, finally, I have nothing left to hide behind.

'Hey, look at this.'

It is a little later and I sit on the floor in my thin dressing gown, my face close to the glass of the holiday lodge patio doors. I have been watching the birds dart back and forth to the bird feeder we filled, and have let my gaze drift to quieter, darker places. Fraser comes and crouches by me, his fingers finding my hair. The new damselfly hangs hidden on the back of the balcony chair, emerald, glistening. Next to it, an inch away, I can see the stiff, deformed monstrosity of the nymph form it has crawled from. It isn't easy to parse the two at first, one ugly, twisted barbs; the other a sleek and certain jewel, and yet something of each is in the other: an echo, a memory.

I watch it for an hour, more. Fraser brings me more tea and affection, pausing to share in my empathy and my vigil. He seems to understand these things too and it makes the whole ordeal one of strange solemnity. As I watch, the damselfly slowly inches away from its old self along the arm of the chair. I had sat and laughed in that chair the night before, not knowing it was there, waiting. Occasionally now, it stretches its wings wide in tested readiness and closes them again. Each time makes my breath catch.

I miss its eventual flight, pulled back into the beautiful distraction of my new lover and our first full day together. I look for it amongst the others by the river later, its green against the usual blue, and convince myself that I see it once, urgent and away. I take a pencil and tease off the forgotten exoskeleton, papery and hollow, and put it in a jar. I feel an affection for it, and envy and resentment, and a kind of protective defence that someone should remember it.

The beds in the spare room stay neat and untouched. We keep the wheelchair and our suitcases in there to mark it as an unapologetic, unnecessary, joyful waste of space.

★

THEN

The doctor had said to stop focusing on myself. He'd said it would help. In the end, I decided that rather than be mad about that, I'd do exactly what he said. It would be a relief. I never liked the story when I was unwell. I wanted to write another one.

I had turned nineteen. My boyfriend was learning to drive and there was talk of a promotion at his shop. I was so proud of him. I still lived at home with my mum and my brother and everything there looked the same as it always did. My bedroom still held its boat, its dent in the wall. The room to the utility room still banged shut when you opened the front door. Mum's dressing table still held her pink roll-on deodorant and a blue tub of Nivea cream. When no one else was in, I would wander the rooms and touch all these things, gently. She and her girlfriend began to talk about the future, and I began to think about mine.

I began to walk up and down our street. I'd set my sights on a lamppost, a wall, a hedge, or a boundary line and walk there and back, past the identical, squat semi-detached houses and their squares of lawn that I had used to skip past as a child. Ten metres one day, then fifteen, twenty, my jaw hard, then back home to lie down, sleeping off the pain until I could go again. Eventually, I made it all the way round the half-moon of our road and saw it as a sign to start speaking my dreams and plans aloud again.

I'd talk about them shyly, delightedly, my eyes shining, to my boyfriend, his parents, mine. In all my dreams, I was well and thriving at last. I claimed wellness as my destiny, swearing I'd do something good with it.

★

I have been noticing old women again lately.

I read these words to him as we lie in bed. Earlier, he had pulled up a chair and read a story to me while I lay in the bath, my legs sharp from our afternoon picnicking down by the river. It was the story of a boy who swallowed a star and I had listened intently as the too-full water trickled down the overflow. Now we're back side by side in the lamplight, I want to read something back to him. 'Read me some of your words?' he suggests, so I reach for my notebook, hesitantly, and I do.

'I've been noticing,' I read slowly, 'that after a certain age, very old women begin to look like stacked cardboard boxes that have been layered with slacks and long t-shirts. Their hips and bottoms square and drop, and they look like they could be unfolded and flattened, or softened by rain. I notice the new position of their breasts, lower, out of the way of anyone passing by who would think to consider them, hanging in comfortable torpor with no work to do. I notice the translucency of their skin and the purple circuitry of them; their thin lips, their flat feet. I notice them because I move like them and share their routines, but I am not one of them. Not yet.'

He is close and listening. I can feel the warmth of him. I have never read any of my journal aloud and raw like this.

'It is the *extra* of them that I like,' I continue, 'at necks and elbows and upper arms; the way their faces hug their skulls companionably. I like the lights in their eyes like an abundance of birthday candles; their long, soft ears.' I hope I get to watch my hair turn white, I say. I hope I am able to start my days like spun cotton, to wonder at the map of my face and think, 'Which way next?'

I tell him, I want a day to come when I will have to stop what I'm doing to remember what it felt like when my skin covered me without a wrinkle and had eager hands upon it. I tell him that I hope that when I do, I will get to hold the pair of hands that knew it then and that they will trace its changed contours with loving recollection, with a different, enduring desire. He smiles at that, the softest exhale on my shoulder.

I say, not being able to stop now, that I want to see what my thighs will do, my stomach, how my tattoos will begin to fold like wrinkled sheets. I say I want to watch the decline of my pubic hair and laugh at myself in a full-length mirror, bold, daring and full of life, still.

'How to hold onto ferocity?' – I have underlined this, for that is what I would like to keep, beyond all. That is what I notice most in the very old women I admire, when it shines from them like a wicked promise. I say, I will shed every ounce of sex appeal if I get to keep something of that.

I chant, quieter in the dark night, his hand on the back of my head, stroking my hair.

It is in the nature of things for me to get old. It is in the nature of things for me to change and wither like a spring tulip. It is in the nature of things for me to lose and grieve. But it is in the nature of things too, I think, for me to leap and win and cackle and make bold, kind mischief until the day I die, and oh, god help me, I want to.

I stop, my words running out, sheepish, suddenly uncertain, my eyes still on the page. It takes an age for me to have the courage to look up at him, his eyes intent, as they always are.

'Oh, you will,' he says, 'I think you will.' He takes my notebook to put on the nightstand and switches off the lamp to draw me closer, to stroke the round stretch of my stomach and pull me towards things that will remind me that my complicated body is still young – deliciously so. To remind me that I don't need to think of any of this just *yet*.

★

THEN

I volunteered one day a week at a local school for children with special needs. Two buses, a short walk from home: I knew I could do it. I helped to take a class of children swimming in the morning and then stayed on for lunch and the afternoon class as an extra pair of hands. I got to know the younger children who moved about their world in different ways; who didn't speak, or who flapped, or shrieked, or rocked and learnt what all those things meant to them. I learnt what they loved and what they didn't. I gave them, in turn, all the love I had.

I was there over Christmas and helped them put on a show; I sang 'Away in a Manger' again, but this time signed the words, the stars in the bright sky accompanied by finger points, open hands. As I got stronger, I began to come back on any extra days they'd have me, and on my twentieth birthday, they sang to me and gave me paintings daubed with red, green and yellow.

Sixteen years later, I see many of them still, grown now, as they attend day classes as adults at my community centre. I spend many mornings writing a few metres away from the room they learn and chat in. They don't remember me, but I remember many of them, their changed faces, their distinctive movements. I remember that you loved Thomas the Tank Engine, I think. I remember that you loved to run in the rain. The first time we met, I thought them to be different to me, but I understand the untruth of that now. I treasure our overlapping days, our joined paths.

One girl of six or seven never said a word. Hers became the face I'd always notice first. I wanted to make it safe for her to be herself. I would often be her carer at the pool, helping her thin body into the frilly swimming costume and threading water-wings onto her arms for her to bob and kick happily in my arms. I remember her rough, dry hands and her unwashed hair, her beautiful, honking laugh in the water like a baby goose. Once, when I was helping her to undress, she lifted her t-shirt to show the delicate pink rose-buds on her vest underneath and with a sudden clear voice and a certain gaze said 'Look!', propelling the word like a slingshot across the room, and I laughed and exclaimed and tried not to cry until the pool water could hide it, that word a new power to us both.

I thought maybe I'd be a children's nurse. I thought maybe it would suit me – something practical and helpful like that, full of heart. I applied and my two A levels and my work experience were enough for me to be accepted onto a foundation degree due to start the following year. I was optimistic that I'd have steered myself the rest of the way towards well by then and applied for part-time care work at a local nursing home for experience and money in the meantime.

It made sense to me. To get better, to fix myself, I would care for people with bigger problems. I would focus on their bodies, their needs, instead of the distracting pull of my own.

★

We get such different firsts, this man and me.

There have been all the usual already. First food eaten in slow, smiling unison. The first awkward pull towards the other: that magnetic ache of distance closing. The first time we realised the relative size of our hands as they found each other – how startling it always is, to see someone's hands close for the first time and to feel them upon you. The first time our lips met and worked out their dance; the way tentative mouths find a beat, become hungry. All the first slow, uncertain touches, first undressings, first gazes with nothing left to hide us. The gasps, like a rip in the air, of first enterings, releases. The first time we did nothing but breathe together. Beautiful, sublime and clumsy, but nothing new for lovers, especially older ones; nothing new for anyone.

We don't get to stay in familiar territory. Our firsts keep coming. They aren't ones you'd normally speak of.

The first time we share a car together begins with his first unaccustomed lifting of my wheelchair into the boot. I watch his arms brace and feel each nudge and thump of the metal on my skin. Our first proper outing necessitates its first inept unfolding and him wrestling with the foot pedals. There follows my first, self-conscious transfer from the car seat to sit in it, blushing, in front of him.

Our first slow journey together is across a carpark, his hands gripping the handles as he worries about his pace and my comfort. I wear a silk scarf that he gave to me on our first day, wrapped loose around my neck. I wonder if I look all right, but then I realise that he can't see my face anyway, so it hardly matters what I do with it. I try to sit tall and not slouch and hope that gives him something.

There comes the first laughed horror at the steep hill ahead of us and the first confident strength of him to get me up it, his breath never changing behind me as he climbs, his hands sure. The first time he reaches to reassure me at a pedestrian crossing – a brief caress of my shoulder, a gentle kiss to my hair, the first close of my eyes to receive them. It is all OK, you see. It is OK when we can't find a kerb-drop and have to go the long way around, OK as we cheer and manipulate our way through a narrow café doorway, tipping the chair up a step, so we can sit and grin at each other face to face once again, holding hands like other lovers do.

These things make me feel more self-conscious than anything else. Even taking my clothes off feels less vulnerable, more dignified, but he is as gentle and ardent in each different moment and there is love, loud and joyful through all of it.

'You look like a creature trying to navigate the wrong environment,' he had teased as he watched my naked, slow, unsteady walk to the bathroom from bed the first time, and I laughed knowing it was true. It is tempting to feel whole only when I'm lying on my back next to him and can make some pretence at being normal, but that is to miss so much of this, and to underestimate so much of him.

There is power in all these different firsts and he sees it. That's the best thing of all – that none of this diminishes, only adds. It only makes love burn in him more fiercely and I feel it. I feel it when he looks at me.

'You know, all this,' he says after another happy day negotiating access and my pain and fatigue, 'I'm grateful for it. It gives me more ways to care for you, more ways for me to earn your trust. It's all just a different kind of intimacy and I don't think many people get the chance at it.' I marvel at him for saying so, for thinking so.

I push myself around the supermarket in my chair in long glides while he pushes the trolley and we debate the food we should buy to share, the noise a clamour in my limbs. We weave down the aisles around the crowds, pulled apart and drawing back as we find each other again, over and over. It is a dance of affirming – my person? my own? – each pull and close drawing the knot of us a little tighter. Everyone around us would think we've been doing this for years. No one would guess the unlikely truth of it.

We lie in the early morning of our last day and talk of it all, of every moment, and he startles into upright, suddenly urgent, and says, 'You know that none of this is conditional on you getting better, right? I don't need that. There are no conditions here.' I swallow back the joy and pain of it against his shoulder and pray that he's seen enough to mean it.

The first goodbye nearly breaks my heart in two. The sun makes the hair on the back of his neck shine golden as he leaves and I put my fingers to it, sealing it like a promise.

A temporary parting is a greater risk than meeting, I've realised.

There is so much more hope in it.

★

THEN

The smell of cleaning chemicals, the ammonia of incontinence pads, the over-boiled offerings of the kitchen: they clung to your clothes, your skin. The totality of it met you like an open mouth when you arrived. It swallowed you whole. To work in the nursing home was like being deep inside the viscera of something ancient, knowing and putrid. We kept it spotless and yet the smell of decay was in everything and everyone and no amount of masking would cover it.

The newly built residential home housed high-dependency elderly patients who all required daily medical care, a great many with dementia and most entirely immobile. You could apply for a job like that with no experience and no qualifications and be emptying catheter bags within a week and that's what happened. Twenty-four contracted hours at minimum wage, with more hours if I wanted them. I learnt how to feed vacant mouths and how to clean dentures and fold nightdresses and pull on shoes around bunions. I learnt how to use a hoist, how to change huge adult nappies when a resident couldn't stand or move and how to wipe bottoms quickly when they could and did. A regular wage meant I had enough to give some money to Mum for housekeeping. It felt like a paltry apology for my still living at home, but it was something. I squirrelled the rest away for university as much as I could and tried not to despair at how little of it there was.

The home's three, featureless corridors made a Z shape and I walked up and down them in my black, sensible shoes with surgical gloves in my pocket, responding to the drone of assistance alarms. I learnt quickly who the good, experienced carers were and stuck close to them. One girl who started around the same time as I did was illiterate and dangerous, another could be rough and impatient, but most were skilled, cheerful and kind. I loved working with them, although there were never enough of us. There was usually only one registered nurse on shift each time who could dispense the medicines and make decisions, and so we did all the rest.

Care work was the hardest, most demanding work I've ever done and I loved it. I came home from my shifts white-faced, wordless, shaking with shock and adrenaline and fell straight to bed, but I felt my heart lift again every time I went back.

★

My suitcase lies on the floor of my bedroom, its contents chaos. I retrieve the silk scarf to wrap around my dirty hair and then take it off again; it smells of another life. I've been home eight days and have been sick.

My doctor tells me I have three different infections: the consequence of being in an unfamiliar place and spending time outside with other people. The consequence of letting my body be bold, too. My glands are like golf balls again, in my throat, under my arms, my mouth full of ulcers. At the doctor's surgery, I stared at the ceiling and past a nurse's ear, mortified, as she swabbed places that a week ago felt bliss.

The intensity of my week has put my body in shock. I have moved about my days shaking with stress, numb to much feeling, and tried to remember what was real. I have tried to be cheerful and present for my son, who knows nothing of romantic love, who I gathered back into my arms when I got back from my trip with relief and with worry.

I have accepted the old routine, done the school runs, weak with fever. I have tried to unpack, to wash clothes, but I can't get the basket down the stairs. I have tried to write and failed and retreated to bed, weeping. Worse, I found that the garden had lost its mind in my absence. Oxeye, sweet rocket, bleeding heart – all had collapsed under their own fervour in a mess of colour. It only made me cry harder. For once, I could see no beauty in it. How to align all this? It is too much entirely.

I have wept for hours. How silly it feels to say it: it was the happiest week of my life and now I can do nothing but cry.

Inevitably, we lost our minds too. We fell out with the strain of it. Accusatory, defensive texts have flown back and forth. He, uncertain that he can cope with such intensity of feeling over such distance, me, half mad with infection, overwhelmed, panicked, and yet soon we fell back together with desperate, ardent new promises. It is calmer again now, rational. We are back to talking of more than ourselves and have stopped behaving like teenagers.

Now, we touch our fingers to the video screens as we did before, full of new knowledge of each other. A mass of white peonies arrived this morning with a get-well-soon card. He has filled my day with gentle words of care, determined to get it right again, to go slow. 'I'm sorry,' we text, in between. 'I'm so sorry.'

We hadn't expected to feel this much this soon, that's all it is. How long does it normally take to know if you want to spend a life with someone? I don't know. It took us five days and god only knows what we do about it now, but he has booked flights for next month. He will come and spend a week with us and meet my boy. That is a start and we will go from there, carefully, rationally, or at least we will try to. We both know the dangers in all this.

My fever has eased today. I go outside, my hair still unwashed, and sit on the low wall of my raised flowerbeds. I try to detangle and stake and tie the plants back into order. I try to remember how to be satisfied with my life. There are more roses blooming than I can count, but how far away they seem. How clumsy and insufficient I feel again; how fundamentally unwell. Bees with swollen legs bob in and out of the bleeding heart. Each plump bloom holds a nibbled, ragged hole at its top, not much larger than a pinhole. I watch a bumblebee stop and test and push her long black tongue inside and the intimacy is too much, as is the memory.

It feels vital now, to have the right gaze on you, to help you remember who you are. Suddenly, I doubt my self-sufficiency. Perhaps that is why the garden collapsed? I spent months whispering to it, telling it of its beauty, its power, its worth, and then I stopped and went away. Perhaps without me, it lost itself in confusion. Perhaps that is the danger of a loving companion as well as its balm.

I must remember that everything has changed and nothing has. I must try and remember how to be alone again.

★

THEN

Life lessons came hard and fast. It only feels strange bathing a naked geriatric man the first time, alone in the huge, sterile wet room. Soon it stops occurring to you to be embarrassed, especially when you realise that they aren't, not any more. I lifted sagging breasts to clean carefully underneath, rolled deodorant onto the soft down of underarms and, without any place to hide or pretend, saw the things that old age does to a body; what it will do to mine.

I learnt with horror all the places that old skin gets sore and tears apart, held bags open for the dressings of abscessed wounds developed during hospital stays on poor mattresses and took deep breaths through my mouth as my heart ached. I sat and pared excrement from under a distressed woman's fingernails and talked in a sing-song voice about everything I could think of as she calmed. I sat with another, writhing and moaning, her back arching as she died and learnt that not all go gently or well.

I washed grey, still hands and faces and helped change the limp, deadweights of people I had said a rosy good morning to only a few hours before, startled at how different they looked with no life in them, learning that faces change without a person behind them to hold them in the right shape. I helped dress them in their finest clothes for families to come and say goodbye before the undertaker arrived, holding up dresses for approval – 'This one? I always liked this colour on her' – a hard lump in my chest.

'You did really well,' the nurse said gently, the first time. I appreciated that. The first time, I went home and sobbed till I was sick, but I still went back. I always went back.

I was overwhelmed and addicted. I have never known a pride like it, not before and not since. This was real work and within the clamour of it, I could disappear. To leave someone's mother, someone's grandmother, clean and comfortable under fresh sheets, smelling of talc with soft lace around her wrists, and to turn off the lights knowing that you have given comfort and care, is, I think, one of the greatest feelings of satisfaction and rightness you can experience in a human body.

I tidied their rooms whenever I could. I read aloud the letters that came and wiped the glass of the photos on their dressers, touched my fingertip to their younger faces in group photos. I spent longest in the rooms of those with no photos and letters at all.

I knew this was real beauty. I wanted it to be my life.

★

It is mid-June now. It hasn't rained for weeks. The grass verges are sickly and yellow. The pavement weeds are usually fierce, filling every finest crack between house and street, pushing through the drains and crowding around street signs, but now they are limp and defeated, crisping into sad furls, brown shadows of themselves. I do not worry though. I know they will endure.

I watch the bared bodies of the mums who share my streets as I scoot slowly behind them to school. Their soft and unapologetic thighs, their strong arms, their round, resting stomachs. My gaze is a long line of stripes and bold prints, last year's summer wardrobe, all a little faded and stretched as we are. Our hair falls loose and cool or sticks in sweaty tufts from our necks and foreheads, scraped into easy care. We kiss our children goodbye; check they have hats, water bottles, sun cream. The air smells of coconut. People everywhere are walking slowly. There is an ease to this faded neighbourhood in the heat and all is unhurried – my pace, for once. Slower things don't pretend and there is a relief in that: a respite.

On my way back to the community centre, I notice that the wheelie bins have lost another shade of themselves in the sunshine. The greens, blues and browns are a little lighter than before; the rubbish in the gutters, too. All true colour left comes from the roses, all else parched. I have never seen such a rampant display. New blooms elbow past the spent, their futures lining the floor in carpets of pink, white, yellow. Very few tend their gardens here and, like the residents, it seems to be the self-sufficient who thrive. Bushes, inherited or gifted, have been left to their own moods. All are out today. All are glorious.

It makes me think of brightly bleached infomercials about nuclear war. I feel like it could all crumble like an old stock cube at the slightest pressure. And yet, there is a strange happiness here, in this bright over-lit world. Thought seems something oddly distant; threat out of mind.

It is hard to let yourself be happy when you know that happiness holds easy traps. It is easy to let fear and doubt and pain wash everything grey. I try to let myself feel it in bright flashes, like sun-flares. Testing, revisiting. I let something burn away.

Too hot to be inside, I pass my friends from the day centre standing and sitting in a circle on the bleached grass under the larch trees at the community centre.

They move their bodies in slow stretches and twists under the sun. It is hypnotic, and I let myself be lulled by it, by all of this. I don't need to hold myself clenched, waiting. I am allowed to trust.

I cherish all of it today, this heavy pause, the pared-back world, our sweaty bodies, while it lasts, while we can. It'll all change again soon enough.

I text him, 'I love you.' That is enough today, I think. To feel it, to hold it, to let it stand alone.

★

THEN

I didn't see it coming. I honestly thought that I'd left it all behind.

Eight months in and my flat shoes started to catch in the corridors until I was dragging each foot from room to room. Nine months, and I began to steal every moment I could to rest, hidden, while my charges dozed in their chairs. It was noticed, of course, my fatigue drawing me into sleep as I sat in the communal dining room, the loaded spoon paralysed in the air in front of a waiting mouth.

Soon, I couldn't lift patients or turn beds any more, not without startled tears at the pain of it and what good was that? I began to phone in sick more and more often, until the doctor signed me off for a month, then another, then another. Soon I couldn't even walk from Mum's car to reception to hand in my sick notes. My previously friendly colleagues turned cold.

I was furious. My body began to feel like something rotten, cursed, and I hated it with dark and bitter resentment while I lay in the childhood bed I'd already spent half my life in. I waited for it to free me again. I'd wake to the sound of the door as my brother came home from college: our old routine. I took up my place as house ghost again. My mother frowned her old, soft frown.

To write it out feels like bad pantomime: 'And then she got sick again!' Perhaps that is why there are no stories told like this, of the roll of predictable, ordinary chronic illness, round and round again. It is so easy to be boring; to feel it. And yet still, I was surprised.

*

I sit propped in the safety of a community centre chair and the open door bends the corners of the local paper with cool air. I am not the only one tired here today. A lady in her seventies, high waistband, chest like soft sand, is slumped and sleeping opposite me, a gold locket askew between the dunes of her. I wonder whose picture it holds; if they are dead or lost.

It is Friday, and that means calisthenics for the Parkinson's group. I play Chopin through my headphones to drown out the pulse of the ceiling fan and the sways of their arms through the narrow windows of the conference room join with the music to make a gentle ballet. I cannot see their faces, just the flow of them, like a wheat field or a slow sea, undignified and beautiful. They will shuffle past me soon and I will wish I could smooth them straight like much-loved letters.

The lady with the locket wears rings on her fingers and a narrow gold watch, unusual in this place unaccustomed to wealth. She has turquoise smears on her closed eyelids and the palms of her hands are pink, scrubbed thin. I stare at the glint of her earrings before my gaze shifts to rest on the pate of another man's head, smooth and shining too, wisps of hair smoothed dark grey with pomade. I admire the respective jewels of them, time travellers to me.

I am glad to be in this world where all can exist as one – my leaden limbs, my buzzing phone, the local news, wrinkled hands and crumpled receipts. I see tanned leather skin; soft bruises and button-up shirts, calf-skimming dresses. I take a photo of my bright pink shoes and send it to my love who knows nothing of this place yet, away in his corporate world of glass.

A man whose jaw shakes veers away from his companion as they walk past, and he lifts the lid on the piano. He plays a dozen notes, waking the sleeping woman with a jolt, before being led away. Another table along, a new baby flaps, arms pistoning up and down in the soft second skin of his baby-gro. Flap, flap-flap. A baby bird, full of flight, and oh, it is so good, all of it. There is much to love here today, and it is love that wakes me up again.

I'm not sure what my role in this life is other than to be a witness. I don't know what my role is other than to appreciate the rolled-open door and the scent of the warm day through it; to watch the tables empty and fill again. Outside, the students from the day centre play swing-ball on the grass, the pole striped like a maypole. If I look up, I can see the tops of the larch trees they play under, restless in the wind.

A new group arrive for lunch, fresh from a meeting in the bigger rooms upstairs. They are suited and hard and jar against the rest of us. They look at me as they approach, at all of us, and their gaze is dispassionate, dismissive. They see a young woman, a little dishevelled, pale, surrounded by the elderly and infirm. They take in my scooter, my slumped comfort with nothing in front of me but a notebook and my phone on a weekday. I see them *other* me, as they other all of us. I see they decide I am not of the real world but something outside of work and purpose and their gaze moves quickly on.

But look, I want to say: I'm here. I'm here to see the man stride past too fast with an unnecessary cane, to watch the tall woman with bruised eyes sip a red drink through a straw. I am here to see you, dressed up in your impassive veneer of professional life and know that underneath, you are just as fragile and loaded with history as the rest of us. I am here, but are you?

Outside on the grass, the rest of the day centre group have gone inside but a young man stands alone and shakes a rainbow parachute into the air. The breeze holds it aloft for one, two, glorious seconds. He lets it fall over his head and for a parallel moment, I can see the stained-glass light from inside it, there through his wide eyes. He's gathered inside by a carer then, body and parachute, and that's it, it's over.

★

THEN

My mum sold our family house; my house. I'd known it was coming. My garage room and its flat roof that roared in the rain, the dining table by the patio doors, the garden paths, the step on the stairs that caught the yellow light. I accepted the new loss as inevitable, with no evidence in my life to suggest loss was anything otherwise. I swallowed it down with all the rest. I told myself that twenty was too old to warrant mourning. I wasn't supposed to be living there much longer anyway. It was selfish to cling to my childhood. I told myself all these things.

It was a happy thing – a new start for my mum and her girlfriend. I told everyone that *it was a happy thing* and wept into my boyfriend's shoulder when no one was looking. 'Please don't leave me,' I'd say. 'Please.' He'd hold and reassure in his quiet, uncertain way. He never knew what to say. I didn't care because he stayed.

I let defiance drive me when all else failed: defiance against all those that were appalled at my mum's new life, and many were. The church had turned on her. I refused to feed any sense that this was wrong, ally and peacemaker as I was, and so I made no room for fuss in public. I was determined to show all on-lookers that I was fine, and then maybe they'd be more accepting. It was too complicated to say, 'I am overjoyed for them and I am heartbroken to leave, to lose this too. I am so confused as to who I am and what is wrong with me and what I'm supposed to do now.' People rarely make time for more than one feeling at once, even though that's usually the way of things. I wanted to keep it simple for everyone, same as always.

My mum's girlfriend's house was neat as a new pin with nothing worn anywhere, and she did everything she could to make my brother and me feel welcome.

Short and wide-smiled, her face open like a child's. She bustled and busied, bright with energy, only to fall fast asleep after every mealtime, her head back, her mouth open. I loved her and have treasured her every day since. We took very little furniture, opting instead for the new start of new things. My sailboat was dismantled and put in the garage and I moved into a double bed made of honeyed oak. How lucky we were now! And the garden! Long and lush, and the house hidden down a quiet road in a nicer part of town, and my mum happy, happier than I'd ever seen her. It made me happy too, but I, betrayer, felt the unbelonging and loss, unbidden, right through to my bones.

I didn't belong here. It caught hard in my throat. I was too old to be living with parents at *all*, but this new time of illness was persisting and none of us knew what to do other than wait and try not to talk about the fact that I seemed to be getting worse. I was lucky, I told myself. Lucky to have them to care for me on the days that were frightening in their severity, even if it was in this too clean, unfamiliar house. I was lucky.

★

I am dusting photographs of my mentors. Four women, unconnected, all in their elder years, all smiling. Each has her own frame on a small table near my bed. I have only met one of them, but that hardly matters.

I have lived apart all my life. I have been hidden and trapped in a place where it has been hard to meet other women like me: dreamers, poets, pounding hearts. If others do live here, then they must have been hidden too and so I have been denied them for the most part. I have had to look for them elsewhere instead, in books, in ideas. I have had to seek them out.

I wish I had known, through the many lonely years, that a coven would form. That it would be made of such varied women, some not even still alive, all strangers never to meet, and how little that would matter to the essential resonance of their place in my life, and to my sense of heritage and connection. I had once missed having God to talk to and imagining His reply, until I realised that there is no need to wait for a divine voice to speak to you when you have one inside you, and when you are surrounded by so many more.

None of the women in my photographs look glamorous and I like that. They are snapshots a loved one could have taken and maybe they did. All own good coats, sensible shoes, and yet they are risktakers, standalones. Nondescript in face, in posture – you'd never guess who they are or what they can do. Their eyes wrinkle like mine begin to. I long ago decided to only aspire to older women so that I'm always steering towards an obtainable future, beauty and poise, not trying to cling to something that time will always leave behind me. Their smiles hide a certainty. I know they would understand me.

Pema Chödrön's shaved head makes her look vulnerable and young and that is apt because she has taught me better how to be those things; how to be open, and to be a beginner, wide-eyed, curious, staying close to delight. When heartbreak came into my life, I bought her book titled *When Things Fall Apart*. Within a year, I'd read all her others. Each one changed me. Maybe this feeling doesn't need to be the end of the world, she says to me from her photograph, challenging, gentle: maybe you could just come back to your day. What else could be true? she asks in my mind when I think I know it all now, and I look again, and I see.

The poet Mary Oliver stands self-contained, her body already turning back to the shoreline behind her, eager to get back to the business of living, and that is right and good too, for it is she that has taught me to trust my body and where it's pulled to, to let its tender form be drawn down, deep into the vitality of everything. Our relationship started with *Wild Geese*, and through her words, she began to teach me how to touch life, and how to let it touch me back, viscerally, intimately, and with unembarrassed hope and joy. It is she who gave me places to walk to when I couldn't leave my bed, as I devoured poem after poem. It is she who has taught me to live with lightness and to be unafraid of death.

Natalie Goldberg looks up and out, grin wide, sensual and confident, pen ready. It was finding her book *Writing Down the Bones* that finally, finally gave me the courage to write what was true. It is she who taught me to leap, to be bold with my body and to dance with life, sleeves up, mind running. To never be ashamed of my muddles, my confusion, the dark compost of me, but to draw it out, stinking and ripe and good, into the light and to smile and say LOOK! Look what we can make with it!

I'm here for all of them, because of all of them. They're how I know the ways to be whole.

Behind them all, in colour to their black and white: my grandma. Not my favourite photo of her by a long shot, but my grandpa stands beside her and a four-year-old me, round-faced in my new school uniform, clutching my orange lunchbox on the grass outside our first house by the factories. It is the combination of these things that makes me love it, need it, in a way that other photos won't do. I am being sent out into life and learning on my first day of school. I know nothing of the world or my future. I wear red shoes, my hand in my grandpa's who holds it gently, tenderly. I stand straight and tall; heels and toes together, smile certain.

I love that little girl, and the woman who stands beside me, her hand unseen on my back, is my courage. She was always bold, self-sufficient and stoic: risktaker, mender, minder. She exudes woman, matriarch and fierce, fierce strength – the kind with no hard edges, no teeth, only gentle hands and boundaries and that tough little push of 'Go on'.

Her memory, since her death eight years ago, has become a flame I hold inside me. 'Grandma would,' I think. Grandma would go for it and hold her head high and move quickly and not look down, not look anywhere except at her mark. And she would wander. She would let herself be free. She would step right over the lines that tried to contain her and she would love who she chose, and she did, she did.

I sometimes wonder if I should add a photo of my mother who becomes more like her own mother every day, and yet I worry to sanctify her here, her and the loving woman she married, as soon as she could, on one of the happiest days I've ever known. I'd be scared to make them sacred – too vulnerable to life's flat foot. Jude would just laugh at the thought of her joining them and would insist on a photograph of her gurning at the camera.

There are others I could add, should add, too. Ursula K. Le Guin should be here. I felt her loss so sharply this year. Reading her books and her sparse and careful writing has given me the confidence to step away from trying to impress and instead to tell the truth in simple form, to let myself believe in the power of words and things and their meanings, to let myself make myth. Tove Jansson, too, who through her Summer and Winter books has taught me that it is OK to be solitary and difficult and how good words can come from that place. Georgia O'Keeffe who first taught me how to look – really look – at the world around me. She should be here too.

The idea of all these women feeds me. Each holds an aspect of myself I have struggled to find acceptance of or a place for. Each of their energies combine in me and I resolve to try and make something good with it. I feel like the uncertain, desperate grandchild of all of them. They form an army of grandmothers I want to make proud. I want to earn my place among them.

I wonder how many more women I will find or who will find me one day? I am not yet forty. God, I always forget that I am still so young. I have so much to learn. I need them to help me and, stuck here, as I've always been, I know the only way to find them is to read and read and keep reading.

That is the door they will walk through.

★

THEN

My brother was to leave soon to go to university. The knowledge of it ticked in me like a clock because once he'd gone, my baby brother, and I hadn't, then I'd know I'd really failed.

One day, I found I'd been off sick too long for the nursing home to have me back and my contract was dropped. I was still a long way from recovery. The dream of a nursing career seemed like an embarrassing joke and I hoped, desperately, that no one would mention it. I quietly pulled out of my foundation degree by sending polite, apologetic letters. Distracted by my illness, I'd not secured accommodation, funding. Every single practicality of what it would take to get me there, for me to thrive there, was laughable – I could barely leave my new bedroom. The shame of it was excruciating.

But if not that, then what to fix my gaze on? What did I have left? What did I have that was *mine*? My fists began to open and close with the need of it.

Start, stop – a pattern had begun. It was me and I was it. A life of constant interruption, I would say, complaining. Whenever I would think myself free and clear of it, I would be brought to a stop again. Back then, I stopped each time I was stopped, waiting to live and try again, not knowing that this still time too was living, that this still time was more real, in fact, than those bright and unsustainable times of promise, laden with the temptation to run clear of myself. I thought, each time that I got sick, that I had gone wrong somewhere and so I threw everything out that had gone before, all that had brought me down — study plans, jobs, dreams, old habits and securities. I did it with a desperate grief, sure it was the only way. I tried to start afresh. Out with the old. Out with me. Try something new.

I didn't know that the interruptions weren't interruptions at all but simply life itself, just as worthy, ripe and portentous with opportunity. I was convinced energy and activity were my birthright. I was sure that feeling comfortable, feeling good, were the baselines and all else an anomaly, and if I did the right things, I would get them back. I strived and planned for *one day soon*, when I would be different, when everything would be different again, when I could try again and get what I wanted this time.

There is good hope and bad hope. There is the kind that wakes you up, inching the heart of you forward, moving you more deeply into yourself, your life — the kind that tells you that you still matter — and there is the kind that carries you away from yourself and where you are entirely. Hope like a secret cold shoulder, a drugged daydream.

'We need our own place,' I said to my placid, patient boyfriend one day at his house where he still lived with his parents too. I begged and cajoled, sensing the rigid noise of his uncertainty. He wanted it too, but his confidence was low, his anxiety high. I believed in him, in us. We could do it, we could, with his music-shop wages and my sickness benefits till I was back at work. It would be tight, and we'd have to be sensible and careful, but there I could get better. There I could properly start again. There, he could grow too, find that new career he dreamed of. I would take care of him, support him, I promised. I'd make it something wonderful. This was the chance we both needed to jump the nest at last. We could do it together! Don't you see? I stayed up late and made budgets and spreadsheets from my bed. I labelled ringbinders and filled them full of long lists of things we'd need.

We filled in forms, nervously. We discovered to our horror that housing association waiting lists were months long, years long, so in the end, Mum and her partner made use of the sale of our old house to take out a small second mortgage, on the condition of a tenancy agreement that would mean we'd cover the monthly cost, and bought a house for us to rent. We found a tiny place a mile away, barely two rooms up and two rooms down, narrow, dark, steep stairs leading between them. It had no central heating and was in an undesirable part of town, but it was safe and strong. A doer-upper. It sat snug against its neighbours on an industrial backstreet that went nowhere but that granted a soothing bubble of quiet. You could hardly hear the main road. The kitchen needed replacing, the bathroom too, but that could come in time. The small, paved backyard, full of weeds, housed one outhouse with an old toilet in it, and another with room for a washing machine. We all helped to cover the walls with woodchip and emulsion, the musty, unlived-in smell slowly fading, dark corners brightening. We filled it full of thin felt carpet and cheap flatpack furniture that mostly fell apart within the year, and I loved it, I loved it so much. The joy of it spread like song. A house! A house of our own!

I had won at last. No one else I knew had a house with their partner by the time they were twenty-one, did they? I said the word partner like a prayer and tried out the word wife on my tongue too, the word mother. Yes. Yes. As soon as I was better. This would be my path now; my road to redemption. *This* would be my own and, this time, no one would take it from me.

★

I could taste metal on my teeth as I scootered back from school, the skies heavy, grey. I think it might finally rain soon but the doors of the community centre are thrown open wide, the fans still whirr.

It's a day you could cut yourself on. It carries rust. I cannot get my legs to move, the pain like an old generator, like a stuffed boiler. I expand under the pressure, perfectly still, the needle creeping up and up into red. I catch concerned eyes today, low and dark as people pass me. The staff keep coming to check I'm OK, bringing drinks to my table. I have crossed some invisible line again. Something about my movement, my sideways slant, is all wrong.

Fatigue pulls across me like a blanket. Sleep, sleep, it says. The temptation to let my body fold and relinquish to exhaustion is overwhelming, but I don't want to sleep. Not now, not now when so much good is happening, when there is still so much to *see*, to learn, to write about. But how to stay awake when your body constantly switches you off? When stupor seems hardwired into you?

If I can just keep my mind steady and alert, I can do it, I can do anything, I know I can. But, god, that narcoleptic pull. I can barely hold my pen today. To lift my coffee is to wonder how anything so familiar can be so heavy. My wrist shakes. I am bone tired. I chant 'Wake up, wake up, wake up.'

It is June the twenty-first: the longest day of the year. A large group of women are doing yoga on the yellow grass outside, lithe and taut in their leggings, like birds in a sallow lake. I crept past them on my scooter on my way here and managed to heave myself into the waiting armchair, trying not to look at their perfect, harmonised warrior poses.

My back to them, I close my eyes to remember the things I've seen this morning. I noted them as I passed them, curating them into a list with each new addition: new tethers to the day, to keep myself awake. There were baby blackbirds everywhere, pecking at dry bread left on a scrubby verge, their plumage jet now but their beaks still brown and nondescript, unthreatening to territorial males. A mother with a wide behind and cracked heels pushed a pushchair and sweated through her top, herding serious-faced children along the pavement. They all stared at me as they passed, their heads turning one by one in a line. The clover was flowering, victorious in the drought: tiny white pincushions tinged as with blood from pricked fingers and yet soft and yielding. A flock of doves flew overhead, turning in formation, grey and silver and white, like pennies falling from an unseen hand.

Blackbirds, mother, clover, doves. I chant my list. I breathe. I try to hold fast.

I shouldn't be here today. I am eating cafeteria food I can't afford and achieving nothing and yet I stay here because I am lonely and afraid.

Why can't I just be happy? Why is it so hard again? Perhaps I thought I'd become someone different now, now that I am newly loved, newly challenged. That I'd float up on the joy of it, up and up, above everyone else, and from there, look down, benevolently, escaped, words and inspiration pouring from me like clean water into the world with nothing in the way. Perhaps that's what feels so sharp today: that I'm still here and still can't.

I am tired of failing today. My work, my life – it doesn't feel like going slowly in this moment; it feels like failing. I avoid my house like a terrible secret, like a truth I can't bear. I wonder what it is. Fifteen years, I have lived there now. I have grown it like a great tree around me and yet to be in it right now makes me itch. It makes me want to scream. I ignore the inevitability of having to return to it in another hour to rest. Yes, often I long to leave, to move on, but where else could I go?

'It all feels so fragile,' I say to Fraser as he calls me before bed. The pressure, the pulse of my pain and anxiety makes me worry I will break something. I know I could.

'It does feel fragile,' he says, 'and it is teaching me so much about you, about us, about what we need.' Who on earth says these things? He does. His voice is impossibly gentle. I rock in my bed in the dark once we've said goodnight, in trust and in hope.

I can only be of use to any of it if I let myself be here, still and calm, awake to what passes. I must try not to throw any of it away just because I am uncomfortable, however tempting. How easy that would be.

★

THEN

The cheap red sofa in our tiny living room was already covered in stains. I put a throw over it, but our cat clawed at the threads until that looked worn too. I'd sit on it, my sore legs stretched in front of me in an echo of times past and try and make something good from each day.

It took three years to recover this time. For two of them, there was no improvement at all, whatever I tried – and I did try, and try, and try. That's how it was supposed to work, right? Effort in, improvement out. But only later came the slow creep, creep of progress, and even then, it was hard to see.

This time, I spent most of it entirely alone, unable to leave the house I had claimed as my victory song. The was no mobility scooter to free me back then, no babysitters to lay out crafts on the table, no family popping back for lunch. My boyfriend left for work long before I was able to get myself up or dressed, my limbs useless for hours. I'd listen to the sound of the door thumping closed and nine hours later, hear the key in the lock. The sounds formed a parenthesis around my days. I'd lay out the things I'd achieved in the interim as if for assessment. Some exercise done – walking practice along the street again, even if it was only twenty steps – study for a distance learning course, a book read or eagerly highlighted, some housework done, a cross-stitch picture finished. Each formed my commitment to wellness, to activity. I'd dress myself and get up and go downstairs, the steep stairs a new mountain, even if it took hours. I was not giving up, see? I held it like an animal in my fist.

He came home from work each day, exhausted. At weekends, we'd visit his parents or mine. We watched a lot of television. We lay next to each other companionably at night and avoided touching one another, at first because it hurt me too much; later because we lost hold of how.

I don't remember much about what we talked about over the years: I remember instead the things we skirted around, the wide and sucking holes. Perhaps we talked about the things we watched and the easy gossip of the day as we always had, our many worries, the many things we wanted, the many things we had to do without. I believe we'd have struggled to articulate much more than that back then, even if we'd had the courage to try. We had neither of us learned how to hear any deeper truth yet, let alone how to give it honest words.

★

Ready or not, he's coming. He's coming to see me again and I haven't changed magically in the interim to become someone different, better. Did I think I would?

But then, but then. He's here and there is joy. Oh, the unexpected deliverance of it, that he should come and there should be nothing but joy after all.

My son adores him. I knew he would. They have been corresponding for weeks too, exchanging words, pictures, gifts. He arrives laden with toys. 'Benefits of the job,' he says, a little embarrassed by his own exuberance but hungry to share. He steps quietly into the air we have prepared for him as if he's always been here.

Our first evening together I spend bookended by both of them on the small sofa watching a film, our bodies squashed together, a hand in each of mine, and it is so perfect that I weep in quiet, smiling streams, my son turning and grinning and squeezing me tight, understanding after all.

There is room for all of it. Room for my struggle to get up the stairs once it's time for bed – the first time he's seen me tackle stairs! – Fraser's careful hands behind me, steadying, as we laugh at the extended view it grants him of my bum. 'How can this be a bad thing!' he grins as he helps pull me to standing from the floor at the top, an ache visible in his face as he draws me close. A kiss to my forehead that pauses: 'I'm sorry. Jo, I'm so sorry it's hard.' Ten minutes later, we are reading poems to each other in the lamplight and there is room for that too, oh yes. Room to move on.

I show him shyly around my neighbourhood. I bring him to the community centre and fail to write as he sits in the familiar chairs and writes in his own notebook, his fingers smudged with ink from his fountain pen. I am learning that they're always like that – a deep bruise on his index finger, his thumb. He keeps a journal every day, dozens of volumes piled up behind him to mark his life. All I can bear to do when he writes is to sit and study the sight of him, dark glasses perched, his left hand scratching the sprawling details of his days, knowing now, believing with new trust and desire, that this is a sight that I will come to know as well as my own handwriting.

He walks the school run with us, past the mothers and their lines of chicks, smiling as we call our usual greetings to our lollipop lady, waving to my son's friends and shaking their hands, their faces awed. 'That's the man who works for LEGO,' they whisper, the news having shot round my son's class as soon as I told him. Fraser's hand is back in its now familiar place on my shoulder as I sit in my wheelchair in the playground, his fingers reaching up to brush the nape of my short hair, and I feel him shake, with both loss and redemption. He had once wanted children, but life said no. That is a colour to all this I should share.

The night before my son's birthday, we wrap presents and blow balloons together, both grinning at the new territory. 'Me from a year ago would have questions,' he keeps saying, shaking his head, enchanted, profoundly surprised.

He meets my family at the party – all of them. My mum and my step-mum, my dad and his wife, my brother, my Jude and her husband and all the children, and my ex-husband too, and his new wife, and his family, and everyone. A tenth birthday party is a good opportunity to go all in, and he takes a deep breath and embraces it. It is as if all time collides. It is a bell to ring out what has been and what we are now and what we could become, all division and conflict past – here, here, glory be, glory be, and peace, peace abundant.

It is over too soon. Fraser and I prepare to say goodbye again, enraptured, holy in this new love. I have no fear of separation now. After these days together, there is a new understanding of what this could mean for our lives, without a need to doubt or grasp or want more. We lie together through our last night, gripped close and marvel that we found each other, eyes wet, mouths wet.

I let myself feel every shuddering, miraculous breath of it, unafraid for once and, perhaps for the first time in my life, not greedy for more. I give it all I really am. I let myself trust. There is no rush.

We will go to see him in Denmark next, at the end of the summer school holidays. The prospect of flying, of all the assistance I will need is like a rollercoaster scream inside me, but I am here for it. He wants to show us his world too. And why not? Why not, now I know anything is possible? Besides, we will deal with me being unwell, I know that now, because this is a happy story. It always was.

★

THEN

Through the years of my slow recovery, my symptoms were severe enough for the doctors to find new interest in me. When I didn't get better, I went back to tell them: that's what they tell you to do, and so I did. My difficulties with movement, exertion, sensation and bodily control were unusually pronounced. Suddenly, the doctors began to talk of hidden diseases – the rare and peculiar, the often missed. Lupus, endocrine disorders, genetic conditions – my consultants proffered new words to explain what might be happening. I was ushered back into the realm of legitimate disease, ferried back and forth to appointments in the wheelchair we'd hired from the Red Cross. It took me days to recover each time.

I reached for each explanation like a cursed prayer. I didn't want to hear the answer, I didn't want these things, but I did hope, I couldn't help that. I thought a name for what was happening might at least mean treatment beyond anti-depressants and painkillers – a plan, a support system. I'd spend weeks convinced of resolution. I'd feel some lightening of reprieve as the

people around me seemed, finally, to believe there was
something to blame here that wasn't just about my
weakness but rather something they could treat, or at
least manage. I would take either, I would take anything.
Yet my mouth felt full and dry, full of new fear: I didn't
want to be sick. I wanted to be well. But, then, the new
ground would fall away. I'd be left numb and confused
when, inevitably, the first-line scans and tests came
back inconclusive and my formerly passionate doctors
shrugged and discharged me. 'Chronic fatigue,' it was
concluded again, and that was that.

When diagnoses or treatments are ruled out,
your pain stops counting. It's a matter of resources,
you see. There is only so much sympathy and time
to go around. When I repeated the symptoms and
experiences that had resulted in emergency referrals
months or weeks before, doctors now listened with
pained, uncomfortable endurance as they flicked
through my discharge letters.

I was asked again and again if I was depressed,
anxious, but I wasn't particularly. When I looked
at the list of criteria – sleeping all the time, trouble
concentrating, moving slowly – I felt confused. Did this
mean I was depressed, or was this simply a description
of profound, physical fatigue? But when they asked
me if I still took pleasure in things, I was able to say
yes, yes, and mean it, and so, in the end, mental health
treatment was deemed unnecessary. My body was

overreacting, but my mind didn't seem to be – I was managing my mood, my behaviours and my thoughts well. My cheerful and practical nature began to feel more like a curse than a boon. A psychiatrist was seen as 'over the top', waiting lists already stretched by people with bigger and more obvious mental distress than mine, so I was never referred to one. More than one doctor asked, exasperated, 'Look, what more do you want me to *do*?' They didn't want to continue dealing with me as a physically ill person, but they didn't really have the time or resources to consider me as a psychiatric case either. It would be easier, it was made clear, if I would just go away.

Hope began to blur with fear and with a deep, abiding shame. They muddied until I couldn't tell one from another. I felt so guilty that I had put everyone through this yet again when I had sworn I wouldn't. However hard I tried to stay sensible, rational, it felt like my fault. I should have been calmer about it all when I'd got sick again. I shouldn't have gone to the doctor and wasted everyone's time. I should have just ridden it out quietly and not made a fuss. I'd only done it to be responsible, I'd tell the doctors through tears, but tears only ever made it worse. You're supposed to be responsible, right? You're supposed to make good decisions about your health, to report the ways your body isn't working, to resist putting your head in the sand? To seek help? I had tried to do the right thing. Please, I promise, I'm doing my best.

They said I would have to try and live with it all as best I could. They told me I should be glad I didn't have a horrible disease. I was, I insisted, I was.

When new discharge letters came, they always mentioned if I'd cried. It wasn't illness or the lack of one that the doctors seemed to object to, it was the fact that I had feelings about it – as if feeling itself was the disorder.

★

It is proper summer now. I want to shout it. Not just dry, but hot, hot. The July air is thick enough to have a scent and to be outside is to be gripped firm. I feel held upright. Enveloped by it. At the community centre, I sit at an outside table for once next to the bleached patch where the lawn had been. The doors are open, the air desiccated, the sky grey and cloudy.

The grass everywhere is white and sallow. I have never known such drought. I took Fraser to the graveyard last week before he went home – the largest expanse of grass I know – thinking we could picnic there, but it was like bone, breaking under our fingers, our resting bodies. I cannot tell you it was beautiful, the lake low on its haunches, the sun too bright, the air too quiet. Another time, perhaps it would have filled me with despair, but how could it then?

'What if *we* caused this?' I had joked, stretching out my arms to the ruin, and then wanted to cover my mouth at the words. Do I believe in that kind of balance? That to receive something so glorious is to drain the world of something else?

I have thought about it since but no, I don't believe it, I don't. I believe that is a convenient lie we're told: that joy is a commodity, that it is sparse, and that is why we must desire and buy and clutch at it with greedy fingers, tight enough to make it bleed, and envy anyone else who seems to have it. It takes brave eyes to stop looking at your prize long enough to take in more than you, but if you can, you soon see that the whole idea is wrong.

A fluorescent badminton net has been strung across the community centre grass and my disabled friends are hitting rallies with unexpected precision. They are not the only ones out here today. An old woman from the sheltered housing complex, thin and bent with snowy white hair – she is out here too. She scampers on the grass with stiff little leaps and jumps, clapping her hands, like a wicked pixie in a fairy tale. 'Dance!' she calls. 'Dance! Dance!' And the little dog around her feet jumps too, pushing to its hind legs to scamper with her, pink tongue long and happy.

You see? There is joy enough. There is joy enough for everyone, abundant wells of it bubbling up through this plundered land, from beneath our dry feet. Let us not doubt it for a second. Let me not doubt it most.

★

THEN

Sweet girl. There was so much I didn't know.

I tried to make it right on my own, the way I always had, back on the red, stained sofa. I turned twenty-three, my boyfriend twenty-six. Mum and my step-mum took a deep breath and borrowed more against the mortgage to have central heating fitted, the bathroom done, worried about us making do without. As I was too unwell to clean, the house was always grubby. It began to fill with cheap purchases we couldn't really afford. Things we clung to, if only to give life some colour, our credit cards too tempting. Our boredom, our disaffection, our need for entertainment, piled up around us, bright plastic stacked high. Good days followed bad days and bad days followed good. I fought against the tide of it.

I read everything I could find on unexplained chronic pain and fatigue, on CFS and Fibromyalgia and all the other names that are given to these things: dozens of differing opinions and studies. Each presented their own explanation for why I was the way I was. I didn't want to rule out the idea of somatisation either – that this was all the result of some hidden distress, my body trying to keep me safe – so I bought the books mental health professionals recommended too and did all my homework. I read up on health anxiety and Cognitive Behavioural Therapy. I crafted new, stricter pacing schedules, special diets, gentle but determined exercise programmes, new relaxation and meditation routines, ways of monitoring thoughts and feelings, of relating to pain – new things to lay out to show for my day. I read books on philosophy, Celtic and pagan spirituality, social psychology, alternative medicine too, thinking that if I didn't hold the answer, maybe something bigger than me did. I'd spread the books and exercises around me like a summoning circle. The four walls of our tiny house became prisms of focused intent and I burned in the middle of them.

They could tell me I wasn't sick in any way that really mattered to them, but they couldn't tell me I wasn't trying. This was my comfort. This was my atonement for being such a monumental pain in the arse. I would *make* myself well and leave this behind and then everyone would like me again and I could stop apologising to my boyfriend who'd come home from another long day at work in retail, depressed and disheartened.

Without experience or confidence to know the good advice from bad, without insight to recognise what I was doing or to see the sucking, poisonous beliefs I was feeding, I floundered, grasping, gasping for some perceived kind of wholeness. I would pull at something and when that didn't seem to work, when I didn't feel better, begin pulling at something else. To look back is to think of a boiling pot, all swirl and disorder.

I didn't know that rain and fertiliser were the most helpful tools, so I reached for a rock hammer. I only knew the sharp kind of being, and so I bashed and bashed at myself, desperate for change. I didn't know it had to happen slowly. I didn't know that I was already whole and contained worlds aplenty. I used all my fire to bounce from jaw-clenched, lively determination to frustrated despair, and, in the end, I blamed myself for everything.

I was at war with life, convinced it could be tamed – that I could be tamed – convinced it was all about feeling better, having more. There wasn't a wise little voice to listen to because they'd told me that inner voice lied.

★

I am in bed again, watching the clock until it's time for school pick-up at 3 p.m. I am thinking about the tumbling of walls and the building of them. I am thinking about cages. I am looking at my familiar bedroom that needs repainting and tracing the black line of mould that runs around the broken seals of the window.

The school holidays start tomorrow. I do not know how I will manage them; they demand more than I have spare. There is an extra physicality to the holidays that pulls at my guilty desire to give my son the fun and play he deserves, my inevitable grief when I have to say, again, no, I can't, I'm sorry, as I try to hold life together from my bed.

I worry about too much screen-time and inside sloth as we wait for the weekly help from my mum that will mean we can go somewhere else, when from the edge I will watch them and other families enjoy themselves – *real* families, I'll think, despite myself. I worry about the extra money that I will, inevitably, pour out on trying to ease the difficulty of it, when I can't make meals, when he is bored and I am eyes-closed worn.

I know the lure and lie of *the only one*, how easily I could use it to convince myself of the things everyone else has that I do not. People have always told me to think of other people who are worse off, to give me some perspective, and yes, that's important and it helps, but I have learnt a perverse trick. Instead, I lie still, and think again of those who I believe to have more.

When we are sick or held back, we talk of being trapped and deprived. There is devastating truth in it. Difference is real. Choices are limited, sometimes impossibly so. We don't all get the same and it isn't fair. I used to seethe and despair at that, especially when others didn't seem to appreciate it; when they didn't even seem to realise how much more they had, but I rarely stopped to think what all this 'more' added up to; why they didn't. 'I would be different,' I'd say, until I stopped.

When you are plucked out of the race, you get a chance to know people because you have the time to look at them properly; their lives and minds, their choices, their patterns and ways of being. I have learnt to study other people as well as myself.

Slowly, I have learnt that for everyone, safety and security are fragile. I have learnt that human minds are not a natural place of peace; happiness and pleasure are fleeting. I have learnt that the very nature of existence is not set up for human comfort. None of us is free: we're all in a cage, each one of us hurting and wanting, each one of us afraid of loss and pain.

Some people have far less than they should, while some people have far more than they need, but this idea of you and them, it's a mistake. It's a misapprehension created by our fear, our disappointment and the brutally unfair systems we live in.

I see it now: everyone around me is full with desire, no matter how much they have. Wanting, wanting something and not getting it. Wanting to be well, wanting to be loved, wanting to be safe, or valued, or happy, or a hundred other things. When things don't feel right, we are all pulled by the idea that now isn't all there is, it *can't be*, and our eyes fix on something different. Especially if now hurts, but even if it doesn't. But! But! But what *if?* When things do feel right, finally, we want to keep it that way, and when, like water through our fingers, it starts to ebb away, we look up furious, despairing, deciding what and who to blame. Everyone around us misses things right in front of them as they play out these patterns; you do, I do. Much is lost in suffering.

It still isn't fair. It still isn't *just*, but in this hungry place, irrespective of our different bodies, our different lives, our humanity joins us. Viewed through this lens, there is no you and them, no in here and out there, only us, and the walls we build around each other inside this shared predicament; the walls we build around ourselves.

I am exhausted today because I've spent the last few days pulling together my finances for submission. I must lay out what's come in, what's gone out, so that the government can decide whether I still qualify for financial support. The weekly Tax Credits I receive hold my fragile life together and I am grateful for them every single day, but I know they could be taken away at any moment. I must still, repeatedly, prove that I deserve what I get.

People have spent my whole life building walls around me based on who they think I am, what they think I'm worth – walls of financial entitlement, or lack of it; walls of legitimacy, help, opportunity, judgement, care, freedom. The walls they build have eaten into my life in very real ways; they have pushed against my body, my strength and my resources. They have tested my capacity to survive. Their force grows more year by year as powers-that-be redraw their opinion over who they think deserves what, cages of fear and want closing tighter.

It has been in my anger at this some days – my honest, mouth-dry *fury* – that I have seen it most clearly: that I do the same thing to others. I draw lines between us. I ascribe to them my own assumptions of freedom, feeling and deserving, deciding what they have, what I should have, weighing the scales. I assume I know best how life should go. I draw out territories, claiming what I feel is *mine*, convinced others have no knowledge of it, that they couldn't possibly, like a teenager muttering that no one understands. I feed this way of thinking about humanity, about myself. It eats into my life, closing me further in. It eats into theirs. Each time I turn away, in quiet bitterness, in righteous surety, I reinforce the system.

Not all walls around me have been built by others. Some I have built myself, brick by brick, unknowingly yet with such sure determination. As I've grown and learnt, I have pulled some walls down. Others I've needed help with, needed love. Other still won't budge and stay beyond my power. In amongst them all, despite them all, I am learning how to be free, and how to create freedom for others.

To cheer myself while I rest, I decide to tell others on social media about our trip to Denmark next month; I speak about my new love. 'You are so *lucky*,' they reply, they stress, and I can feel the jab of their finger as I scroll through their responses, the pull of their own desires and pain. I hear the unspoken questions, the whispered accusations: 'but I thought you were sick?'

I am lucky, I say, I reply simply. I know I am lucky, and I look down at my body that I now need to get down the stairs somehow, to haul it onto the scooter and, for the last time until September, to school and back, and my mouth shuts tight.

It would be so easy to be resentful and defensive. Instead I blow on the blinkered, frightened nature of such statements, knowing I have made countless myself. I let them collapse: a wall made of sticks, that's all it is. All that's left is to smile with understanding at the ridiculous, narrow-minded predictability of our perceptions. Not everyone else has my pain, but all around me have their own.

I focus on the smallest next step. From my bed to the landing, that's all I need to think about right now.

That's how everyone must live, regardless of what they have and have not. All of us must still make one next step and then another and try to choose well, try to choose bravely, try to choose in a way that pulls the walls between us down and throws cage doors open wide. We must do it so we don't waste our lives with wanting or grasping or trying to avoid pain; so we can all know what it means to be free in a society that doesn't want us to feel it.

Time to face the school holidays, then. There is no need at all to build more distance between me and everything else. Life is hard enough.

I swing my legs off the bed and begin.

★

THEN

When I wasn't trying to improve myself, I would dream. I dreamt like an addict, drawn back to bed to let my inner stories unravel for a little while longer.

Lying still, eyes closed to the world, I hid fantasies that I'd play out time and time again, shaping them, colouring them, feeding them, telling myself that by doing so, I was helping to make a better life, a better me. Desire is the first step in getting what you want, my books had said. Picture it. Visualise yourself well and thriving. Visualise who you want to be. I had no idea what a powerful, dangerous magic this could be.

At first, I practised ready for my big moment of emerging from what I had and leaving it all behind. How easy it was to grow it bigger, bigger. Different lives. Different selves. I began to fabricate houses, routines, famous friends. I rehearsed thoughts and words, scenarios, practising, willing. In each fantasy, I was special in some way. In each I was *chosen*, plucked from this life and into a new one, by someone, something. I had always been able to step into my head and away and now I did it with an adult compulsion I couldn't shake, my mind fixed and greedy. Soon, I let my dreams bleed into my waking day – a constant, background movie-reel of other.

I have few memories from that time. I lived mostly in my head – walls within walls. I rarely looked up at what was really there. I rarely looked out. I never spoke the whole truth to anyone. Perhaps I was frightened to do so, the grief and confusion at my lonely reality too strong. I retreated into my imagined lives. I assembled visions of what I thought might make me safe, whole, worth something, and I fled to them at every moment I could. To admit to what I was doing would be to admit how unsafe I felt, how unloved, unworthy, and that seemed like a betrayal, so I never said a word. Instead, I'd press my hands to the growing ache and gnaw in my belly and imagine it swell. A new wanting. Oh, an indescribable void. Yes. That felt like the answer.

I began to say less and less again. A smiling mask returned: a placeholder until I could become what I was meant to be.

I wasn't depressed, I was a preta — a hungry ghost. Fill me. Fill me up. *Choose me*, I begged of life, please. News of a schoolfriend's wedding would send me into weeks of bitterness, the envy and impatience like bile. The pregnancy announcements were worse.

I dreamt and waited for my boyfriend to ask me to marry him and wondered why he hadn't.

★

I take a deep breath in and out again, my heart full, the screen propped against a pillow on my bed. I change my mind and shift myself over to the mirror to apply some more mascara first. He'd laugh at that, but a girl's got her pride and the skin below my eyes is dark and swollen and I look too tired without it. I have looked forward to seeing him all day. My son spent the day refusing to settle to anything I suggested. 'I'm bored,' he'd said a dozen times, grumpy, restless. 'I'm lonely,' I'd hear.

I have felt very alone too. I press Fraser's name and see *connecting* . . . and feel a little faint. I still do, every time.

When Fraser first suggested that we should switch from our back-and-forth written accounts to video calls, I was amazed to find I said yes. I have said hello and goodbye to entire relationships without often talking to them on the phone. I have avoided spoken conversation about myself like a cursed thing, bolstering myself before any exposure to it, using listening as a way of hiding. Deep down, I have been sure that if I talk, I will get it wrong, that I will break something, and people will hate me, leave me, hurt me.

While many things have healed and changed, this has lain locked. I don't often have the confidence to say how I really feel. It is a button done up in my throat. I feel it there, hard and choking, and I can't undo it to say the words I need to. I can write truth, but I can rarely speak it aloud, not often, and not easily. I struggle even with Jude, with my family. I can't do it without going home afterwards and shaking and feeling sick, not without questioning every word that escaped me and wishing I'd never said a single one, vowing to speak less. It is no way to live: an old, old reflex that life hardwired in.

And for all this I said yes to this man I hardly knew when he asked if we could talk over video. And he, almost as resistant to conversation as I am, he asked the question. Our desire to learn more about the other overcame our habit to be silent. We make a baffled, antisocial pairing, and yet we find we can talk to each other. We find that, despite ourselves, we answer the curious, longing questions of the other.

Because these times are scheduled, limited, we put away phones or other distractions when we talk. Sometimes I knit, but mostly, we simply sit, one body to the other, and look at one another, a wide sea between us, finding the words we want to say or have saved up since last time. Some weeks, for long days, I am not well enough to lift my head from the pillow and so he must see me like that, but we said we'd talk every day and we have stuck to that, no matter what the day has brought.

We've talked about how hard we find it to be emotionally honest with other people – that conversation was a miracle all its own. We've agreed that these calls could act as a commitment to a new, honest intimacy with each other; a vow of care; a resolve to not make *this* relationship more complicated than it needs to be by hiding things from each other. We've agreed to make it a safe place.

'Hi!' I say, still a little shy.

'Hello!' he says back.

'How was your day?' we both say at once and laugh.

He talks of office politics, of the neighbourhood cats, of how he's washed and waxed all the floors of the house, even though it's another fortnight till we arrive. 'I think I'm nesting,' he says, embarrassed.

I talk of my son, how I was spun today from deepest, aching love at the sight of his bare knees in shorts and his devouring of sandwiches, to desperate, suffocating claustrophobia. I talk of how we sat and decorated letters from a craft kit I'd ordered – J, K, F – an initial for each of us and how they now hang on the window. Fraser looks away automatically, his face flushing with delight, and then he pulls his gaze back to mine, smiling, to tell me how much that means to him.

I feel it rise too as we talk, just as I know he does – that buttoned-up-tight feeling of danger, danger, too much, I am saying too much and it will spoil everything. I pause, gather myself, and speak through the tight sensation. He was brave enough to. I can be too. Back and forth, slowly, we let the day tumble out. I talk about my writing and how the words felt today, about my desperate desire to learn and improve. He talks about a forthcoming work trip and how much it helps to have me in his life, how easily he can feel untethered. One day, we will need to talk of harder things than this. I know how much this daily practice will help.

There has been another change. I have learnt to smile with my mouth wide, my teeth bright. I have only smiled like that with my son before, behind our doors, not ever with another adult but I cannot help it now – my careful, closed mouth has been left behind. My joy at seeing my new lover's face each night has drawn it out of me.

'I missed you,' he says, suddenly. I cannot help but beam at him. I draw a finger along the line of his jaw on the screen.

We smile. We chat until we begin to yawn. We slowly learn to talk aloud our days. We gently learn to talk aloud our fears, our shadows, our hearts.

★

THEN

One day, in the last days of winter and the first of spring, I was sure it was time. I had not long turned twenty-four. My birthday had come and gone. Valentine's Day had come and gone, and nothing had happened, so I had orchestrated this drive to the forest. Snow fell gently and we walked a little way in our usual stilted but familiar silence. My determined walking up and down the street had begun to pay off again. These last few weeks had been easier, and I thought he might say it now, with me walking beside him. I knew exactly how it should go: the snow falling, him falling with it to kneel on the melting flakes with a ring long hidden in his pocket that had been waiting for just the right time. We walked the path by the trees slowly. My heart beat like the rock hammer. Almost back to the car, I panicked. 'Don't you think we should get married?' I remember his blink, and the flush of his face, nervous. After some stumbled words he agreed, yes, yes of course we should. He had been waiting for me to get better, he said, but yes, I was doing a bit better now, wasn't I? It would be all right now. He said it with love.

We drove to town and chose a cheap ring, anxious about the money. I made him do it properly then, already rewriting the whole experience in my head to make it sound more romantic when I told everyone.

'And a baby? When we're married?' I asked, my womb like a squeezing hand. I bought a big binder and a stack of glossy magazines and started planning. It was the happiest I had ever felt.

I'd sit in my bed, a hand on my stomach, my hope something hard. Smiling, wishing, willing, avoiding the quiet man in my house.

It is easier to see now, at least. It is easier to see now and so, this time, I can try to go a different way.

★

It is dark. I can do nothing but lie still.

My head pulses. I must keep my eyes closed, even the softest brushes of light causing me to flinch and retract. The exhaustion has me bound tight. I can't lift my legs, my arms, my hands. To make them move I must haul them, like wrecks through heavy water. Standing brings a trembling and a vertigo that leaves me gasping. It is a black sea to be lost in. The pain that accompanies it is an all-consuming bite.

My breaths come ragged, torn, and I must focus on keeping the keel of me steady enough to contain them. When I move, I hear hollow moans from faraway and know they come from me.

I must drink. Water helps, but I don't know how to get up to fetch any. Did I eat when I got home? No, I didn't. I made my son something with his help. I crawled to bed as he ate, pulling myself up the stairs on buckled legs, pushing strength into my arms. I have been here since.

We went to the zoo for the day, that's what we did. My mum had a day off and my brother came too; his strong hands to push me, his warm humour to lighten everything, my son bobbing lovingly at his side, taking photos of everything. There was laughter and love and joy through all of it, and I was careful, too – elevating my feet in the car to stave off the pain that comes if my legs are vertical for long, stretching gently in my chair to keep myself from tightening. And still this.

It is hard to reconcile this as anything but punishment. It is hard to find a way to think about it peaceably, positively, when it feels like such a living nightmare. There have been nights like this when I have been sure this was about atonement – a balance sheet I could never repay. There have been nights like this when I have wanted to die, but not for a while now and not tonight, and I am grateful for that.

I try to use my training. Pema would tell me that pain isn't punishment just as pleasure is not a reward. I detach, I step back, just enough to observe sensation's movements, its ebbs and flows, rising thoughts of panic or worry touched and allowed to move away as I stay close to my breath and my body. I know that this is nothing dangerous and nothing to worry about but even so, I am a woman alone in the house with my child, unable to move, in enough pain to find it difficult to speak, to stay silent without that low, instinctive, animal moan, and that is a hard thing to be. I do not want to overshadow the day, to drown out its glory, but I am here now, and I am suffering. I'm allowed to find it hard.

So extreme the fallout. How could this be right? And yet, it has always been so. This is not an unusual place to find myself in. Days of far less activity have resulted in it but I have a tendency to forget in between. I believe it is too much for my mind to hold preserved and so, each time, it lets it fade. The brain does not retain the memory of severe pain when it has ended, mellowing it, distancing it. It does it to help us go on.

I decide to fetch water. That small step can be my next decision tonight. My son is asleep now, having got ready for bed by himself, unperturbed, used to me saying, 'I need to rest, love. I need you to help.' His

A STILL LIFE

lack of alarm at the severity of my state was a grief in itself.

The trip to the bathroom will mean more pain. I breathe slow and calm to prepare. I am trying to sink into kindness. This is a hard thing to experience but I am OK. This is not my fault. It is not anyone's fault. Being kind to myself will help. Water will help. I am safe.

I manage to pull myself to sitting and then standing with a little cry, eyes closed against the vertigo, my heart instant in its gallop. One step moves forward a little easier, the other drags behind, and one hand holding the glass, the other on the wall, the door, I lurch and creep my way down the landing. It is five metres, that's all, and it takes me an age and I hear the dragging sound I make in the dark and let out a rough laugh despite myself, at the night-time monster I am.

I get there at last and fill the glass, letting myself notice the space around me as I have learned to. The rough woodchip under my fingers on the wall, the blue glow of the window, stammered in its cut glass, the glint of the mirror. Peace, peace in my house, and I try to let it fill me too, broken as I feel. I am peace. Peace is me.

I drink some there and refill before I make my way back, step by step until I'm in bed again. I let myself lie in the resulting storm of it, filling my head with soothing words as the pain rises like a wave and hits the rocks of me hard. I am OK. It will be better in the morning. There is no sadness and no fear now, I am simply sensation itself for a little while.

Exhaustion pulls me into blackness time after time and I let it. When thoughts float back, I turn them into healing words. I focus on bright images from the day. My son's laugh. The face of my mother.

Life is good. Life is good. I choose it again and it is worth it. I say it to remind myself. There is more to me than this night. There is more to all of this than I can see right now. It will be easier tomorrow, a little at least, and more so the day after that, but in a wave of shifting physical awareness, I feel the familiar pull of my bladder under the tide of pain, my control already giving, my underwear already wet, and I let out a sob despite myself.

This is a difficult night. Sometimes you just have to say that too. This is not an easy life.

★

THEN

The day came that I gained a new room in my life: a library. It stretched up cold around me, its radiators smelling of dust, distant ceiling tiles thin and loose. The tall bookcases that filled the room reached only halfway up the smudged cream walls and were made of hard mahogany. The books themselves were greasy and worn, the paper yellowed, cracked spines all in a line. On the quiet times no one else was there with me, I'd breathe it in and out, running my hands over the wood. I'd worry sometimes that I'd get caught, sitting there, smiling at the empty, waiting chairs, at the neat box of tickets, happy tears in my eyes. I'd open and lower the metal blinds with a rushing clackaclackclack and laugh, wincing.

I *was* feeling better. The weeks before our engagement hadn't been a fluke. It had taken a long, long time but something invisible had turned itself. I used to be sure it was all the work I'd done on myself – that's what I'd say, that it was because I'd worked so hard.

I still walked with a stick, but that spring and then all through the summer, I found that I was well enough to get out of the house by myself for an hour or two, to walk to the bottom of the road where there was a gym with a pool, to do aqua-fit and yoga, and sometimes, sometimes, make it to the graveyard, with its views over marshland and the sound of lapwings and geese. I laughed loud again, full of joy. I sparkled the long-awaited ring on my finger. I felt like I'd been given a new chance at life, at becoming who I was meant to be, and so I had immediately done what I had always done: I had applied for a job.

It was perfect for me – a part-time position starting in September, running the high school library at my first high school across town. I would work the afternoons as part of a job share with the senior librarian, a few hours a week. The library was scruffy, old and under-resourced – just one big classroom – the pupils more 'challenging' than ever, as they warned me, but more importantly, it was on the ground floor, and once I was in it, I could stay put. It would be just like old times, I joked!

I'd arrive at lunchtime and be the last to leave, the cleaners nodding their hellos as I made my slow way back down the corridor, my pace picking up month by month until I no longer needed the stick. I barely saw another adult apart from the occasional teacher who would pop their head around the door or teach a class there and so I never made friends, but used to solitude, I didn't mind that. Besides, I was rarely alone. The children came and went in rhythmic droves. I collated a group of waifs and strays who would gravitate to my desk at every opportunity and find excuses to stay after school. Shy children, needy children. The too-thin, the always-dirty, the bookworms and the anxiety-ridden, the unwell and dysfunctional. I took care of them in a way no one had taken care of me back then, when I'd been like them. I listened to the complicated accounts of their lives and read them stories aloud with every bit of energy I could muster. I started bookclubs, craft clubs, comic-book clubs.

I began to say that I *had* been ill but was better now. I ached and got tired, but I was sure it was just the last vestiges of something leaving my body. The long years stuck in my house became a story I would tell of the past, rich with my victory. I *used* to be in wheelchair, I'd say, but I'd fought my way back to health. 'Look at me now,' I'd smile, taking a firm step away from my past self, like a mean girl from school moving away from the unpopular kid in the corner. She wasn't with me.

My engagement ring caught the light. I talked about my approaching wedding with the younger children who drank up every word, huddling round the photos I brought in of me at my dress fitting, the pictures of the venue, the flowers I had planned, and they cooed. The walls slowly transformed under the colour of my displays. I gleefully organised and rearranged and ordered new, exciting stock to tempt in the teenage readers and soothed the ruffled feathers of the older librarian who had been used to doing things the old way, who would come in each morning to find more changed.

It was a happy place. I had so much to give them. What I'd once poured into my care at the school, at the nursing home – what I'd later pour into my parenting – I poured into them. Warmth and care streamed from me, something unlocked, until I got home.

More than one door shut behind me each day. Back home, I would be kind and affable. I would try to listen to my fiancé's days, his worries, try to support him through his work and concerns, but it all felt strangely distant. I would find myself awkward and clumsy around words and feeling, a wall in the way of the easy attention I could give, should have given. What *was* this?

We never talked about it. I used to wonder if he even noticed. I noticed though. I berated myself for it, sure it must be yet another of my flaws.

★

We are at my mothers' and I have wilted after dinner like I often do. I have gone to lie on the grass in the shade of their garden. They have brought cushions and made a bower for me amongst the flowers. I lie back in it now, the pulse already receding from my legs a little, the hot, thick fog in my chest and my throat and head already easier to see through. I rest and look.

The green around me is a visceral shriek, almost unnatural in its brightness. Bright orange lilies push against the blue over my head. The hours my mum spends watering every day have sustained a richness here that I haven't seen in weeks. I have to keep closing my eyes to the over-saturation of it, pain thick, breath slow.

I will have to pace it out. I open my eyes for a little while then close them again. I see what changes.

I watch goldfinches and long-tailed tits shoot back and forth across the sky. When my eyes close, I can still hear them, over that pulse sound that summer makes, which I wonder if others hear as well. Is it a thickness to the air that I can hear? That I feel an echo from? It is something in the sunshine, something in heat. It pushes against me, unquestionable sensation, and I know it because I am all sensation too. It is not a soft pulse of growth, not like spring. There is something sharp and predatory in it, but here I know I am safe.

The breeze weaves through the long, ornamental grasses, through the damson trees, a few purple thumbprints of fallen fruit already in the grass. I let my toes find the sharp edges of blades of grass that have turned hard and woody in the drought. I watch the cabbage white butterflies that seem to have been everywhere this year float past me in ones and twos and think of my Fraser, turning to text gentle words of belonging and to receive them in return.

I sleep. Body heavy on the earth, I let myself belong to that too for a little while, to be broken on it and to heal, to float on sunshine and quiet and bird call and words of love, and the happy movements of my family on the patio. I rest on it all.

I wake to the hushed word, 'Mummy?' and murmur a greeting back, his long body dropping and extending to fit behind mine, his nose between my shoulder blades, his sticky fingers finding my arm. We whisper words of assent and enquiry and he fidgets, and I hear the sound the air makes just before he smiles, out of sight behind me. He is happy.

We roll onto our backs and watch the clouds, impossibly white today against the blue, and he tells me in a long stream of confidence what he sees – a dragon, a plane, a fish – my eyes still closing and opening like the butterfly's wings. I smile and agree, one finger tracing circles onto his waiting palm. This is our secret code of 'everything is OK'. He smells of sweat and oranges and youth. Our twinned bare legs fit next to each other, the hair on our arms overlaps.

How can a ten-year-old have learnt so well how to love? How can it flow from him so easily? Like sunlight, there is no effort to it, no thought. We move together like the clouds do, without needing to make a single choice. No agenda, no concern or doubt, no worry. Love like air around us. Love like peace.

A stir in the stillness and he is gone, calling his plan for what's next back behind him as I listen to his feet thump on the flat lawn. I lie in the aftershock of it, the breeze finding my untouched skin again, my mind clearing to new awakeness, and I know then that I have known true love in my life; that for all the other times I have squandered it, misled it, I have at least been with it now, whole and present.

I want to put my hands to my chest and hold it there, like a saint in a painting. Knowing, enduring.

★

THEN

How to talk of relationships that died? Tiptoe around them, or drag them out into the light? I don't know, but I know there is no use pretending we lived happily ever after. I can't write as if we did.

I remember so little of our time together through those years. So terrifyingly, blissfully little. I remember the sight of him getting dressed in the morning, cheap trousers pulled over the dark hair of his belly, shirts tucked in, his face newly shaven, pink and ripe like a pomegranate. I remember the fluff of his socks on the bedroom carpet and hanging them out, stiff, to dry. I remember folding his t-shirts into careful squares and leaving them in a pile on a chair.

I got my dreamed-for wedding in the May after my twenty-fifth birthday. I had spent over a year planning it and it was as beautiful a day as you could hope for. My bouquet was peonies and daisies. My new husband was handsome, ardent, and as I said my vows, I didn't want anyone but him. Our family and friends surrounded us and spoke of how we were meant for each other, how wonderful it was to see me looking well. I smiled the whole day, even when it poured with rain as we raced to the car to take us to our hotel.

I woke the next day, empty. We drove to Scotland for our honeymoon and lay apart each night and every night. I barely spoke at all for the whole two weeks, numb, deeply in shock. Shock at what, I didn't know, but it was physical and real. If he was confused, he didn't say it, lost in his own thoughts.

I did love him. Oh, I did. I loved him with the easy, blinkered, needy love of childhood – the only love I had known. I knew nothing of union or compatibility then, nothing of partnership or the necessary roles of solitude and self-reliance within it; knew nothing, even, of romance or the fever of it. All I knew was love brimming with anxiety, with dependency, full of a need to belong to something, anything. I loved from that shallow place and thought myself full because I didn't know what full felt like.

I loved determinedly and fearfully, without insight or honest communication, without any understanding of the passage of time. I loved with a real and genuine longing. I loved with a beginner's love.

Back home, we settled back into our routines as if nothing had changed. My new husband began to volunteer at a youth centre in the evenings and we spent more and more time apart. The mundane days alone felt like a game I had to play. I tried to make the right moves so life could work out the way I wanted it to, and the abiding, awful horror of it is that I was convinced that was all there was to it.

And a baby! How could something so perfect come out of something so confused? And yet it did, our son did. There has never been a moment's regret in that.

A baby will fix it, I thought. A baby will fix *me*.

★

I am reading again the way I did as a child. I lost that ability for a while. I was only able to read in short, furious sprints before distractedly turning away. I worried something had died in me, but like a seed, it had simply lain dormant. Slowly, it has grown back. Now it is unrestrained.

I had forgotten the mad trust involved in giving yourself over to reading, in opening a book you haven't read before and saying, 'Right, so we don't know each other, but here I am and I'm fully prepared for you to change me entirely, or not. Whatever. Let's go.' I had forgotten how much it is like true love. This is why readers are dangerous and extraordinary people to know: they have mad trust running right through them. They've honed it with every new read. This is why, if you don't feel very brave, you should read more books. They are why, I suspect, I had the courage to fall in love again the way I did.

I wonder whether it is something about trust that is allowing me to read this way again. New trust is growing in me, and where once I would have sat and fretted or poured words and attention into internet black holes or quagmires of thought, now I sit, calm and self-assured. In that space and stillness, it is easier to do nothing at all and instead reach for a story.

I must let myself go to read. Perhaps that is what I have been missing – that mad trust to abandon myself for a little while. You can only do that if you feel safe in your body. If you feel wrong, the panic and drive to fight and control yourself hold you back. They hold you tense and watchful, like sitting with a snake in the room. It is trust then, trust in ourselves and our place in the world, that we need to read well. Only then can we let ourselves go and know it will be fine.

It is another day when everyone around me sweats and fans at the air. I am in my usual chair at the community centre. Every window is open, every arm bare. I sink into a winter land of snow and fur and I am there, utterly, for a long while, crawling along the ice sheets of a distant planet, my eyelashes crisp, the ground creaking like old wood.

When the spell breaks and I look up, I am amazed to see my own arms bare too, warm and pink, and to realise I am not cold. The sun beats down on the parched grass outside, the way it has done for weeks. I am struck again by the freedom of letting my body be in two places at once, living two lives. And because

I am whole and at peace, not grasping for the real world to affirm or punish me, or the imagined world to rescue me, I can move freely between the two and become something new. I can see. I can *learn*. I can let myself be both people, each knowing exactly where and who they are, where they join, where they don't. This is what books have taught me, more than anything: that there is more than you can see. That there is so much *more* to all of this.

A book can sit on your shelf, unread, underestimated for years, and then when you finally pick it up, you find it changes you. It was always going to, one day. You can live with yourself in much the same way.

I must keep reading. I must go everywhere it can take me, and I must do it from this gentle, strong place. Where I'm not afraid to let go. Where I'm not afraid to come back.

★

THEN

I lay on my back with my bottom on a cushion, my legs in the air against the bedroom wall, wondering if this would be it. They told you to do that, after sex. Tilt your pelvis UP and raise your legs, to increase the chance of conceiving. I had read all the books, all the magazines. The wall was a dirty blue and needed painting – the cheap woodchip scuffed and marked, pictureless. We never hung many pictures. Our wedding pictures stayed on their CD.

The business of getting pregnant felt formal after so many years of us lying next to a different kind of wall. A wall for my legs, a wall between us in our bed, a wall in our talk. But we both wanted this baby and our shared joy at the double line on my test a few months after our wedding was real and loving. We were always better friends than lovers. That was good enough for a while.

My belly swelled, imperceptibly at first, until it finally looked how I had pictured it through so many of the long days I had lost myself to fantasy, but the sensation was beyond imagination. Finally, I was awake, *here*. I felt ill every day in a dozen different ways, horrified by the monstrous helplessness of it and yet newly alive. My old limp up the corridors to the library slowly became a waddle. 'You're getting massive!' the kids would say, astonished, impressed. We'd sit around my desk and watch my bump through my t-shirt, waiting, waiting, until it came. A PUSH. A kick. 'This is so weird and brilliant,' a boy told me, his eyes wide.

My body held. Although I was forever sure it would fail me once and for all, it held firm through this changing. It made me feel powerful as well as afraid. The ferocity of it was more like righteous anger than the resplendent peace of the fertile goddess I had imagined becoming. It made me want to defend, to move, to make noise, to retreat. A growl. A bite. Not out of grumpiness, but from a haughty, unshakeable alertness as I held the world together. I felt animal, and not tame.

A son. We were to have a son. I felt our boy grow. I felt him stretch and roll. I'd stroke the hard line of his spine through my stomach. We bought a rocking chair, ready. I'd sit in it and sing to him, read to him, and the love and fear that grew was beyond words, beyond what I knew I could feel.

With nine months' readiness came a sinking knowing. I'd feel it like anticipated trauma – a thickness in my mouth. This would not save us. It would not bring us closer, my husband and me, now there were two of us where once only I had been. There was no going back now but I knew I'd never have chosen differently, whatever the truth. I'd always have wanted any path that led to this.

Now there was my baby and me. We were joined in a way I had not known I could feel with another, and as my son, sticky and bawling, was placed in my arms and I bled half my life out into the hospital bed, I wanted nothing but him.

★

It has been years since I have flown. I had forgotten the sensation. I had thought that it would feel like what it is – like flying – my body weightless, effortless for once. I imagined I would become like something of the wind for a little while.

Instead, I feel reforged inside the tight aluminium. I am earth and rock. I am a whole new planet. My legs have turned to fire and cooled to iron. I can feel the thrum of the pressure and the movement along every fault line, agonising and vital. Outside, there is only blue – deep atmosphere cobalt fading to gentle, smudged cornflower, a white line of cloud brimming the join like a horizon. I hurtle through it. It is glorious.

My son is at my side. We held hands as we took off and now let our arms rest against each other as we relax into our separate sensations. He feels it in his ears, he says. I feel it in my everything. We mouth simple, happy things to each other through the muffling of our headphones. I had forgotten, too, how noisy flying was: another trick. Looking up at planes passing overhead, I had pictured easy silence in this empty space – the silence the birds know – but humans and their machines, not meant for these heights, can only roar with the effort and gleeful audacity of it all.

I can't do a thing. My eyes are fixed to the window, my heart full of awe at the sky and at myself, full of love for this eager chick at my side. We made it through the airport thanks to his determined care. He had pushed me in my wheelchair possessively, refusing the help of our assistant except for the trickiest parts. As I stood to walk the few steps down the aisle to our seat, he stayed close, bracing himself to take some of my weight, determined to help, darting back when I was seated to make sure they folded up my chair correctly, the air stewards smiling.

It is not a long flight. I don't need to worry that it hurts, or that I am tired. Knowing it won't last long, I can put it all aside and let my head lose its strength and simply sink into the wonder of it, the companionship of this brave thing we are doing together, my boy and me. We catch our courage in our words and our gazes at one another and pass it back and forth. We both know that this is the greatest kind of adventure.

I watch each thought as it passes until there is no thought. I want nothing in the way of this. I want to be all here, knowing that is the best gift I can give.

We will land soon and Fraser, who has been crafting this trip for weeks, will be there to scoop us up and carry us to rest. He has filled the footwell of his car with cushions so I can relieve my legs and sleep until we're home. He has placed powder blue hydrangeas and glass lanterns on the doorstep to welcome us in, filled the cupboards full of food, the vases full of flowers. I know these things but I have not seen them yet. The expectation that I will, soon, keeps pace with the thrum of the plane. I will gather him in again too, care for him too. I can't wait for it.

I had thought my body couldn't do these things any more but here I am. I look around at the other passengers, all different, all carrying their own fears and flying despite them and I am proud of the lot of us, one and all. There is another woman in a wheelchair on this flight. I watched the tight muscles of her limbs shake as she transferred to her seat, her daughters clutching soft toys and bright bags, all alive with chatter. I know we are both teaching our children not to be afraid. I know, too, what a privilege that is.

I will be exhausted for days, I know, but it doesn't matter now. It is better to be alive like this, stretching, seeing. The relief that I am still willing to try is like the cool breath of wind I had waited for, and I feel myself lighten after all.

★

THEN

For a while, I was sure I could still take care of them both – my husband and my son – and I wanted to try. But as our baby grew clever and sleepless, full of colic as I had been, and often, it seemed, utterly furious at being alive, I was drawn back and back to him, to soothe him, to feed him, to show him this bright world.

My world shrunk again. I was twenty-six. I had left the library, my job there ending at the end of my maternity leave due to more government cuts. I said goodbye to the children and promised to visit. My family all worked long hours: Mum trying to avoid redundancy, my brother beginning teacher training. My dad's wife had left him, suddenly, and his answer was to move further away, to throw himself into thought and places that didn't remind him of the past. I understood that.

My husband and I made good parents, gentle and patient as we both were, but he was still mostly absent too, away at work each day as he'd always been, the click of the front door still bookending the hours. Needed as I was, endlessly, I pushed our spindly, quiet marriage further and further from the nest to make room. He offered no resistance. I'm not sure he knew how or if he would have been able to.

I'd walk into town sometimes, leaning on the pram, but tired quickly. There was very little sleep, and breastfeeding came hard at first. It was easier to stay at home. New baby groups offered friendships, everyone bright and willing. 'You should go! It'll be good for you,' people said, when they thought I was spending too much time alone. That's what they do to new mothers – rope them together until they Make Friends. I'd sit on the hard chairs, bouncing a crying baby on my knee not knowing what to say. I could never quite blend in like the others. I'd get close enough then feel it like sheet glass. I was just out of practice, I'd reassure myself, and try to ignore the familiar, quizzical look in their eyes, the half-smile, the tilt to the head. I tried to ignore the old heat of it.

I began to write then, for the first time. I was so full and so isolated; I couldn't think what else to do. It didn't occur to me that I would be good at it, or that I would try to be.

Out it poured. I wrote of this new love I had found, the shock and splendour of it. Of motherhood, of abject exhaustion, of the bad days of pain that felt like a foreshadowing and made me worry about relapse; about the days when I thought the demand and sensation of all this would swallow me whole. I wrote about how lost I felt and how found. I described my growing boy and the things we learnt together in our solitary days; about anything that wasn't my husband, or my failure as a wife.

The love I felt was staggering. It was what I had long needed – divined, somehow, and steered towards. Adult, responsible, clear-seeing love, terrifying in its truth. Fierce and responsible, knowing and brave. Love that looked out. Love that didn't look away. I knew I would do anything for it, for my boy, that I'd let anything go to see him soar. The shallow-rooted marriage that had given it to me smiled sickly in its shadow.

★

The skies are so big here, my eyes can't hold them. I must turn my head as I sit in the car to catch it all, as we drive over the vast bridges that join the land together. The weather shifts and deliberates even as I watch it. Black cloud to rain to bright sun, as if its attention is caught and its mood altered over and over. I see something of myself in it. I want to open my arms to it, an empathetic sister, and when Fraser drives us to a sheltered fjord beach, the car only steps from soft sand, I do.

Denmark is a quiet place and it suits me. It spreads out around you, flat and green. Each neat, low building politely draws a little apart from the next, freshly painted in reds and blues and greys. The roads stretch to the horizon, long under beech and pine forests that pull your gaze edgeways into a distant, soft darkness.

I do not feel afraid here. Fraser's care is so immediate, so solid, that I can rest in it and open. He helps me to the water, and I sit on the damp sand, pulling off my shoes, pushing red toes through the line of seaweed to let the tide lick at them. I sit there for a long while. I notice everything, letting my gaze rest on one thing, then the next, then the next, staying with it just a little longer than feels natural, sealing each thing.

I begin to fill my pockets as I sit, reaching from my centre point to turn and gather shards of mussel, shattered quartz, the smallest, smoothest pebbles of orange and yellow, bleached cockles and fat whelks, even a curve of white sea glass. My two join in, roaming further afield to bring back oddities for me to bless, my obvious joy like a hand upon us all, the sun low in the sky, the waves full of spilled light, pouring itself to my feet.

It is a perfect moment. Brief and absolute in its contentment. I do not try to explain or justify any aspect to myself. I do not grieve what isn't. I do not try to leap from it hungrily into elsewhere or try to hold it fearfully still. All simply is.

What a rare thing that is. Horrifyingly so.

Contentment is mostly relief, I have realised. It means you can rest.

★

THEN

I do not know what happened to start me dreaming again. Perhaps the intensity of motherhood had eased ever so slightly, just enough to offer me the space to lie still, alone and undistracted. Perhaps my son's naps grew just a little longer. Perhaps I'd never really stopped at all. The old question was right there waiting for me in the long hours until my husband got home – 'But, what if?' – and I reached for it like the old addict I was, grateful for its familiar touch. You're supposed to think big, aren't you? You're supposed to be ambitious. Opting out was a sign of disease, I knew that's what they'd say. It showed you'd given up and I was never going back there, where they suspected that of me. I must keep moving. I must outpace the fatigue and fear always biting at my heels.

The internet only fed it. I had discovered social media during the long afternoons breastfeeding, the early, sleepless mornings. I peered in at other lives, greedy for new things to learn about the world out there, about anything outside this house. I found it ripe with things to admire and envy. In the same rooms I had once dreamt of the fidgeting baby in my arms, now I dreamt of new things. Not fantasies now, but practicalities. *Sensible* dreams, I told myself. A new house, perhaps? A bigger one, with a proper garden. A better neighbourhood? A proper career? Other people had these things, why not me?

I had started sharing my writing on a blog and to my surprise, people noticed it, noticed me. I began to be offered things: opportunities, press trips, praise, respect! Paths I could walk, people I could meet. Tantalising things. I'd roll them around my mouth like a new taste, sweet and comforting. These people didn't know that I was nobody. They didn't know I was a failure. Could this be my future? Seen? Admired? Chosen after all?

I saw the way people online talked to each other, the way they wanted to talk to me, the things they talked about. Nobody in my real life talked to me like that. I wanted it: the stimulation of it and the belonging. I wanted to run to where they were, somehow, and feel my world expand. I longed to be challenged, pushed, to be stretched until it hurt. Years of clinging to safety and now I wanted to push it as far away from me as I could make it go.

And, sometimes, quietly, carefully, telling myself it was only daydreams, I began to dream of passion too, of the heat of desire, the wet and greedy suck of it, of what it might feel like in my body. I'd think of it with my baby on my lap and burn with shame but still drew a little closer to the thought. Like roots reaching for water, I felt my mind probe. I'd imagine a different face, different hands. I'd feel guilty to have even thought it, afterwards, when I was pulled back to my life, but I told myself I was silly to feel bad. It was only natural to fantasise. Everybody did it! What could be the harm in it? The change in me happened so gradually that I didn't see it. I didn't feel the water heat up around me.

I didn't want to be small any more. I didn't want to be *minimal*. I felt indignant anger.

'I didn't know!' I wanted to shout at everyone in my life. 'Why didn't you tell me? Why didn't you tell me I could have all this?'

★

I can smell the apples that surround me. One more hits the floor with a thump every few minutes like a slow, irregular heartbeat. I am lying under a blanket in a hammock strung on a heavy frame on the grass between the trees in Fraser's garden. I lie with my ear against the day and listen to the life of this new place. The blue sky and its racing clouds are above me; the apples in the trees like green moons. Every few minutes, I hear a flutter and imagine I can feel it on my skin: a sparrow beating its wings in the branches. I watch the blue tits land on the feeder to turn their inquisitive heads with an alarming twist. I worry they will fall to the ground like the apples.

Fraser's garden stretches wide and bare but for the three old apple trees on the lawn. Each one is full, aching with the weight. The windfalls make a haphazard, pockmarked circle around each tree, as round and broad as each canopy; two red circles, one green. He picks them up sometimes, in a burst of resolve, filling a wheelbarrow, and piling them behind the shed. He stands in the evening and admires the smooth, uninterrupted expanse of the lawn, but by the next morning, the circles have returned, perpetually renewed.

We pulled out the hammock, full of apples itself, so my head wouldn't be in the drop zone as I rested today while Fraser went to work, but a small one has landed on my feet and I am surrounded. Come autumn, he tells me that he will climb a ladder and pile what's left, ripe and unbruised, into boxes for his colleagues to bake with until even they tire of them, before making a mountain of the remainder by the shed for the fieldfares to feast on all winter. Hundreds upon hundreds of apples, high and green and red and fat, and dozens and dozens of birds, giddy on the fumes. I am looking forward to seeing that, I tell him. We have already planned for my return.

It is cold, the season turning. How strange it is to be somewhere else. Our house back home, the community centre, my little cage of streets – they feel a long way off. Can that really be my life?

My son is inside, safe, happy. Fraser will be home soon, and then, I think, perhaps we will drive to the beach again or to the supermarket, or light a fire and play games until bedtime. We are having to make a lot of time for rest while I'm over here, but none of us has minded that. I have been very tired, and we've had to go slow, but we have each been content. It has been good just to be together, opening to each other. Soon we will have to say goodbye and I will go back to my solitary life for another few weeks and my son will go back to school. It is hard to want it. I am already conscious of the hungry desire all this has woken in me and I watch it like the goshawks we pass as we drive around this new country, sitting silently on posts at the edge of the forests.

We began this week playing at being a family until we realised we were one, are becoming one, blushing like the apples. To be out together, to be *three*, joined and loving, under the gaze of other families, accepted as one of them, has been a startling new energy.

It has been simple things that have caught us unprepared. Coming downstairs to find the two of them side by side eating toast, playing computer games, chatting without me. Finding my lover's – my partner's – amused, laughing eyes to meet my own, conspiratorially, when my son sulked over some slight, and in that finding a different kind of release; a unity. Shared cooking. Shared chores. Shared plans. Surreal and perfect. New.

Fraser drove us home from a trip into town, my son and I asleep in the car. 'I've never had that before,' he told me quietly, later, as he described the sense of protection and care that was ripening in him. 'It is early days, I know,' we both say thickly, shakily, and yet we cannot deny the feeling of it, the desire to make this our life. To seize a reclamation.

I have denied us this kind of belonging up until now, my son and I, through my choices, my needs, and I will never know whether it was the right thing to do.

The thump, thump of the apples are like truths landing in me and I feel each one. Grief. Hope. With the right wind, there is not much between them. I run my eyes over the windfall. Some are still round and muscular, flexing boastfully at their curves, newly fallen. Others begin to turn in, spreading bruises, bitten with round holes. They sit beside those so far gone, it is hard to recognise them for what they are. They have become withered brown bowls on the lawn, barely apple at all; wrinkled rims and puckered lips, warts and pustules. Wasps and flies pick over these ones most, licking them with their sucking parts.

Suddenly I am afraid to move from this place, afraid to catch one with my clumsy bare feet, knowing it would be pure horror. Suddenly I am afraid to move at all. I look at my skin in the sunlight, smooth and preserved. I want to press a bruise into my white skin until it turns the colour of this unpredictable sky. To have it so unblemished is an unbearable tension.

The neighbour's cat leaps to lie against me in the hammock, her purr a new reverberation. She pushes against my hand, my arm. She stops and begins to make a low sound over and over, hungry, urgent, her eyes on the birds on the feeder, but she doesn't move away from me.

The apples fall, thump, thump, thump. I hear the car on the driveway. I am not going to know if it's too late until I try again.

★

THEN

By my twenty-eighth birthday, I was so lonely I could hardly get through a day. Absences and longing clawed at me, at my throat, my chest – a suffocating claustrophobia. I couldn't breathe with it. It was like a long, slow panic attack, relentless and choking.

I waited to see if my body would give in. That's what they'd led me to believe – that my body was dangerous like that and would betray me at every new emotional upset, but it didn't, not at first. My body plodded on, unimpressed by my distress. I could still get up and move and live and, oh, the perilous freedom in that. Dangerous thoughts could lead to dangerous behaviour, reactive, addicted, out of control. I could do anything. I felt the hunger of it. The temptation. I could do *anything*.

I began to unravel, to withdraw more and more into myself, choice by choice, thought by thought. I'd lie awake at night next to my husband and weep in silent streams, with shame and depression and grief, unable to be near him and sleep, every cell of me pulling away from him. Who even was this man? This stranger? I'd look at him and not know the answer. My words spoken aloud each day became stilted, fewer, careful.

The days passed in numb automation. It was a real and persistent agony and in that there was fear because it felt like death. It felt like a road that led only to death. The threat of relapse flared bright every day. I was terrified my unhappiness would rob me of all my new ground; that the stress would unhook something in my body once more. I couldn't go back there again, to helplessness, to dependency. I would die. Everything good would die around me too. I couldn't let it happen.

My child needed me. It felt like the ultimate betrayal to bring him into this world and love him like this only for me to shrivel and die and I would, I knew, if I couldn't get all this off me, if I couldn't get *out*. This was the dangerous sadness, I knew it. I'd look at my son playing happily with his bricks and cars and quake with terror, remembering a father who had been overcome by feelings like this and had to go away.

I couldn't take care of all of it at once. Not a baby, a marriage and my frightened mind, my fragile body. I just couldn't. There wasn't room. Oh god, oh god, it was going to crush me.

My son turned two. The month after, my husband asked me if I wanted him to move out and I said yes, yes, I did want that. I said that to the man who'd done nothing but his best to care for me and give me what I'd wanted, who'd done nothing other than be utterly, devastatingly wrong for me somehow, for reasons I couldn't explain.

I didn't know how I'd manage, or even if I would, but I said yes anyway. He left a few weeks later, quietly, furious, broken.

I told myself that if it hadn't been me now, it would have been him in a year or two; that if we had stayed together, the gap between us would only have widened until he was driven to find solace in someone else. I told myself that I had seen it first: that this was a young love with no roots and no future, and that I'd simply had the bigger will to face it. More than anything, I told myself that it was better for our boy for it to happen now. We loved him. We would always love him, but it would only be worse later, if we kept dragging this dead relationship between us. I was saving him pain, I told myself. And I needed to be alive, to be free from this desperate unhappiness, to be a good mother, to be well.

I don't know whether any of those things were true, or would have been, but that's what I told myself.

It was the cruellest and worst and most necessary thing I have ever done, and I have never regretted it, not once.

★

Back home, I try to be all here again. It is not as easy as it was.

I survey my own garden like an old cow, my heart pushed up into my mouth. I try not to chew on it, try not to choke.

Everything here is dead or dying. The dry curls of all the plants I didn't manage to care for well through this fierce summer rise crisp and hot, like fires flickering. The soil pulls away from the pot edges, gaping cracks in the desert. All greens are yellow, all yellows yellower. Some things push on, grown huge and frightened with their neglect. They bend low and useless, their too-long limbs scratching at the ground. Bees buzz half-heartedly around the ruin and I want to say 'I'm sorry' to every one I see.

There are moments that no one can prepare you for. There will come times when you must witness the consequences of your own neglect and destruction. You can't always be good. You won't always get it right and you will cause hurt. You will have to stand in the middle of it then, brave and unflinching. You will have to look at it and not turn away, not allow guilt to turn you to stone, or the lure and delusion of an easier alternative burn up all traces of your remaining resolve.

This is not my first time looking at ruin and I tell myself there's no need to be afraid of it now. This seasonal change is how a garden trains us. Pull it back to the brown earth gently, if you must, if there is no saving it. That's where it started. That's where it can start again, and where I can forgive us both.

Autumn

It's happened. I could feel it when I woke up: something has changed. There is a thrum to the air, to the golden light. It is a sensation like the birds in the apple trees. I feel it right through me – delight and melancholy all mixed. There is movement, a tide, a sigh that sounds like leaf-fall. I am not in the same place I was. Nothing is.

There is something in the chill and the sky. It was in the first reach for a blanket last night, in pulling on socks before bed. The rain falls in torrents today and my skin is newly awake with it, newly prickled. Change, change, change in everything, and I feel like I'm spinning; poised on a tipping point, breath held, arms open, heart ready.

There is an itch to pull something out of this feeling, to make something, to prepare. I cast on a shawl in soft, grey Danish wool, watching the stitches march along my needles. I think about my brown boots that barely touch the floor now and stay pristine through each season. This time of year has often brought mourning for their lack of mud and wear but this year I know I can whisper safe promises to them. 'You will see cold fjords and meeting seas, Scandinavian forests, new skies. One day soon. Just wait. Just wait.'

Something in me wants to draw circles on things. I wander around the house and trace them in the condensation on the cold window glass, on my empty desk, on my cheek: one finger, round and stop. An echo of something? The fat, green rosehips in next door's garden, perhaps. A coffee-cup ring, a turning planet, a faded hydrangea's powder puff, an open eye. Wake up, everyone. Wake up! The summer stupor, it's over. We all get to shrug off our bare skins and try again.

September, September. I say it like a prayer. I want to cry it and whisper it: September, September. I want to lie down in it and die a little – just a little – in all the right places.

★

THEN

My boy ran ahead of me through the tall, dry meadow-grass. His toddler belly was round like the sun; his thighs fat and perfect. As he moved, the grass moved with him in a wave. His blond hair matched its colour, and as he turned to watch my slow following, his serious frown held something of its practicality. We were in the field by the Common and the sky was full of the kind of white clouds you are sure you could bite into, if you could only pull them down. I brought him here, out, away, because I wasn't sure I could keep going, but in this place under the wide sky, I think maybe I can. Just a little longer. That's how the days go now.

My new life granted me the full stop I had wanted and was brutal in its uncompromising presentation of that want. I had not really expected to find a reward or ease waiting, but still reality shook me until I was sure. 'Are you certain?' it would say with each new day alone, and then find some way to shake me a little harder, just to see. We talk about leaps off cliffs with images of flight, of soaring; the luck of the wind and the wings of our souls pulling us up and up and on. We don't talk about falling, landing, and what happens then. How bad we are at talking about failure. You can break, and do, but you survive. Often, there's no other way to do it. At least I was awake now. Despite everything, I found myself thankful for that.

When my husband moved out, I had no job, no income. I had told myself money wasn't a good enough reason to ask him to come back, but that resolve was tested with each bank statement. 'Sure?

How about now?' it said, it jeered. 'And now?' I stared and recounted and let things go, one by one. Yes, I was sure.

I had applied for what benefits were available to me until I could work out what to do next. I had first thought I could study, maybe, to try and get some qualifications, but now everything seemed to cost so much and so I simply shrank, so I would cost less. The money paid into my account every two weeks was barely enough to live on, but I'd tell myself that I didn't deserve to have it easy because I had something to atone. I would make it work, I'd say, hard and certain. We'd never had any money anyway. I wasn't accustomed to luxury and I never expected it. Cars, holidays, shopping trips: these were for other people. I'd sit through the Jobcentre interviews hunched in front of whichever smart suit was on that day, braced, counting my breaths like I had used to during medical tests. I tried to make myself small, compliant, grateful. I knew how to do that.

I had never lived alone before. At night, in the bed where once I'd lain awake beside the man who'd felt like a stranger to me, now I lay sure I could hear a more frightening hand trying the front door. I was rigid to every sound. Burglars, predators, worse. They must be able to smell me here, I thought, my baby and I, our vulnerability something sweet and ripe.

'I am brave,' I'd chant in the dark.

'I will look after us.'

'I have done the right thing.'

★

The new term began today. I scooted our old route to collect my son from school – the first time in weeks – and now he walks in his usual place, tall at my side.

A little girl – four, I'd say – walks along the pavement towards us we wait at the pedestrian crossing for the lights to change. She is holding her father's hand. A pink, puffy coat like a cloud at sunset is zipped up to her small chin and around her halo of black curls, she wears a large pair of scuffed silver headphones. The wire leads to her dad's pocket.

She walks slowly, cautiously, her balance thrown by the lack of outside sounds. Her face is a mix of concentration and awe, and aching, wordless pride. Her private smile reaches me as she draws closer, half-focused on her careful procession, one measured foot after another as they come to wait beside us for the lights to change. She looks up and the pulse of daddy's music reaches me with her wide and honoured eyes. She will remember this in dreams, I think. This overlap of worlds from eyes and ears. The first tangible, understood grip of love in her heart, perhaps, and a knowing that this man, for a time at least, this man was the sky.

I look up into his face for just a moment, as we wait. His eyes are dark and tired. I think mine might be too. His eyes flick to watch my son reach for my own hand, and then he looks back to my face. Something passes between us, imperceptibly: a kinship, a knowing. The weight of his responsibility meets my own in the air, and then the crossing lights are beeping, and we turn in opposite directions home.

★

THEN

There were no bright, stimulating relationships to leap into. Of course there weren't. No new life claimed me. Exhausted by the demand of simply getting through each day, most friendships and opportunities I had fell away, or I avoided them, until I barely saw a soul again. A foolish testing of passion with someone I had met online, thinking he might give me something of what I'd craved, fell flat after a few months of sporadic pretending: we had both looked for escape but found only ourselves. I felt the new pain of our tangled remorse. I felt sad to have lost yet another friend. Acutely ashamed of myself, my thoughts numb, I wrote less and less, my popular blog dwindling, dying. Honesty was too frightening for a long time.

I was naive, panicked and deeply, deeply afraid, but as the weeks and months passed, I grew sharp with resolve too. I had made this devastating cut, but I could make sure it was a clean one. It was time to stop falling apart. The damage would stop here, not spread from this place like rot, I swore it. I wouldn't exacerbate it any further through hurtful words or worse choices. I *had* chosen this. It was time to trust that choice. I would make this what I needed, and what my son and his father needed to stay close too. I could do that without being a wife. There would be no war, no winning, and no running away. I'd become an intermediary between them and try to find new ways to nurture what mattered, and for all my other broken vows, this was a promise I kept.

I was often too tired to go out and so we stayed close to home, as I always had. Days passed in a blur of play, domesticity and bright, singing toys. I loved caring for my growing son, and in that lay the secret, in the end. In learning to care for him, in seeing what he needed, I began to learn to care for myself too. We'd sit on the small square of our front room floor watching television and create sprawling, plastic worlds or great ships out of cardboard boxes. We'd walk to the concreted park at the bottom of the road, avoiding the broken glass. We'd paint huge pictures on rolls of old wallpaper – of towns and whales and starfish drawn around our hands. Somehow, often through kindness and sometimes through luck, we always seemed to have just enough, and although each morning I'd hear the letterbox rattle and feel the cold clench of dread at the thought of brown envelopes on the doormat, sure it couldn't last, I felt grateful for each new day that it did.

For all the fear and roar, an awareness grew of something new. I'd catch it in the quietest moments, like a voice in the distance. I listened and listened. Some days, I was so weary I could barely climb the stairs, each movement and moment of care something to be heaved through; I felt it in every part of my body, and yet I survived. An equilibrium was sustained. Some days I was well, some days I wasn't, but I began to learn to let each day be.

I still couldn't seem to do as much as other people, however hard I tried, my capacity bafflingly restricted, but compared to how life had been once, I could hardly complain. I could walk far enough to get us to the park, town, sometimes. I could stand and lift him and play. That felt like enough. Pain hummed in the background like a radio left on.

I'd wake in the morning, early with the dawn and the nonsense chatter of my bright, wide-awake child and try to think, 'Let's just see, shall we? Let's see what this day holds,' and I'd feel new courage in my chest: I'd tackle one thing, then the next.

A gentle humour grew that I hadn't known before. I began to laugh again, often, to smile at nothing and everything. I found delight in the details of our days: in his small socks on the airer, his thick fists around his crayons, the soft brum of his lips as he pushed his cars around the mat and the squeaked, melodramatic crash of his trains. I made a happy, safe home for it all to exist in, however exhausted I was, and I saw how my boy could thrive in it, and how I could too.

My son's growing limbs tangled on my lap as I traced my finger round and round his palm, telling stories, his mouth wide. His eyelashes curled dark and luscious as he slept. I'd tiptoe out, avoiding the loose floorboard and then sit, alone on the stairs, undisturbed with the night. No sounds of parental sanctuary to listen to now, only the gentle shifting of the house, the sounds of my own breath, the drum of rain through the attic hatch. Thoughts came and I looked at them, curious, with nothing left to lose, and it was there I realised I had not been still like this for a long, long time. For all the isolation and time I'd spent cut off from the world, my body holding me back, my mind had only got faster and faster and faster, running and running and running.

In the shock of this new state of being, I finally stopped.

★

My son comes upstairs to show me his new Year 6 topic homework. He has drawn a map of an imaginary Galapagos island from high, high above, and drawn in huddles the creatures he has learned would live there. Here are the iguanas sunbathing on the rocks. Here are the frigatebirds with red, ballooning chins. Here, the Sally Lightfoot crabs, filling the beaches. Here, the giant tortoises, their backs like half-moons.

I let my gaze run over his drawings. He has inked over the pencil lines carefully in pen. I follow a line up across his hands, his arms, to the soft snub of his nose, his still-long eyelashes, his serious eyes. He catches my eye, and I grin, loving and sure, and I tell him it is the best picture I've seen in months. He grins back, delighted. Not one cell of me turns away from him. Not one nerve of me flinches. He sees it and knows he has all of me.

Extreme fatigue brings a guilt with it that aches. When I am at my sickest, decisions must be made. I must turn away from more and more, because any extra will push me further into collapse. I cannot watch the news, go on social media, or offer an ear to a person I know is struggling. I cannot give the world my energy or my time. If I do, I have nothing left for the basics: for homework and bedtime, for dressing and showering. To survive, I must often make the window of my attention narrower and narrower.

Who knows if there will be room for you at the end of it? Do I sound cold? I tell you: it breaks my heart. The memory of what I have pushed away sits heavy. Sometimes it feels like all around me, people are clamouring, clamouring, 'Pay attention to me! Make me important!' and I hear the howling from the world when I don't, each thing and person in their own way, because they needed something I couldn't give. And so, there is left this endless guilt that I am not more, that I couldn't be and can't be more for everyone, because I know everyone and everything deserves care and attention, and I wish they could have it.

There is no use denying the hurt in it. I lost a marriage this way. I know I have lost friendships too. Is this a confession? That I have so often chosen to live shut off from other people so much of the time? That my isolation is as much self-imposed as it is enforced? Perhaps it is.

Today, I must still often withdraw, and retreat and retreat, but, ah, wait, there is a secret. Because now I know how not to close off, not entirely.

Slowly, slowly, I am learning to leave a gap. I have learnt that I can *choose*. I must do it before I'm locked up tight, throwing a shoe in the door as it closes as an act of quiet, desperate resistance. Consideration is necessary because I know now that the problem with attention is that it really can only ever rest on one thing at a time, and that if you don't think about it or notice where you're putting it . . . oh, how easy it is to choose badly.

Each moment then, I choose and try to choose well. I leave room for this one, last thing outside of myself. An inked picture, a play of autumn light, a curling leaf, a face, a run of spoken words. Through the gap of this choice, what's left of my energy and my attention can pour. Narrow, and slight, but all I have, yes. All of me.

Now we talk about the iguanas, the frigatebirds, the Sally Lightfoot crabs. I notice the ink on his fingers and press my own to them. The trick is to let it all breathe without you, and just look, look and listen and love and be there. I remind myself that attention is not about collecting pretty moments to make myself something more, better, or to fix anything – how quickly people use mindfulness as simply another commodity to hoard and accrue and seize ownership of, playing at it like a game to win, a business! No, the work is simply to witness: to let the object of your attention be seen, heard, touched, until you must choose again.

This is sustainable, helpful love, I know that now. I know because I got it so wrong before. Not scattered or pulled about, but considered, self-assured, certain. I can be enough this way, here, with this one thing or this one person or one task, one need. Moments at a time, *I can be enough*, again, and again, wherever I am.

There is grief, yes, for what I've lost and that it took me so long to learn, but the new miracle of it, the dawning magic that I understand now every time I focus my attention like this: I can give small bits of myself away and I won't break again. There will be enough left for me.

Besides, how cleverly love spreads. Even at my most broken now, I watch how the basic, most focused moments make my son grow, and how they make Fraser unfurl too. I see what happens afterwards: they go out and touch the world and other people in ways beyond me. They do good things for themselves. And if I can do that with two people, with a family, how much bigger can my love stretch through gentle words written to others? If I can make you feel something new, what could you do?

From my bed, from my chair, I know that I can grow bigger. I can become a whole house. I may have failed before but now, one person and one moment at a time, perhaps people can shelter in me and feel seen and cherished, safe, and then go back out into the world as something restored and healing, maybe. Maybe they can.

★

THEN

When it was time for my thirtieth birthday, I ran away. I couldn't bear the thought of a party, or even seeing anyone at all. I kissed the round face of my son and delivered him into the hands of his beloved father for the weekend and with hoarded money, flew to Jersey on a cheap ticket, booking two nights in an out-of-season hotel with easy steps down onto the beach. I'd never been anywhere on my own before. I felt sick with the thrill of it, like I'd eaten too many sweets, and watched the dark sea move beneath the plane.

The winter still had its tight hold on the island. The hotel was almost empty and running on skeleton staff. I figured even if I wasn't well enough to walk far, I could sleep here, for as long as I wanted. A different bed. A different view. I brought a pile of books and my knitting.

'Are you here for business?' they asked, as I checked in.

'No, I turn thirty tomorrow,' I said, simply, happily, not knowing why I'd told them.

'And you're here alone?' they asked, confused.

Yes. It was just me, I said, I smiled.

I woke early and pulled on extra socks and hat and scarf and went and sat on the sand to see the sunrise. It pulled itself right out of the sea, red, like something just born, and I watched it climb until it turned into a hot, white star in my vision. I had started taking photographs again, then, and I carried my camera in front of me like a torch. I collected the day.

I did manage to walk a little way, down the dune paths and up, over the headland. I found a bench on a high crop, not far from the hotel. It sat on a circular plinth overlooking the sea, and its dedication read, 'Stay awhile and turn your thoughts to those you love,' and so I did.

It didn't happen quickly. I had to sit there a good long time feeling myself expand and contract like a sea anemone. Pulse and pump and reach and retreat. No, no, it was too much, I couldn't. Until, there, that give, and I opened to it, a sob in my chest.

I heaved up love from every place I could find it in great, wet handfuls. I offered it out to the sea where I knew it would be safe, laughing a little too, at my own passionate, beautiful absurdity. I gave my broken marriage, my son, his father, my parents, my brother. I gave the gap where friends should be but who I didn't know how to hold. I gave a new man I had met but who I didn't know if I should see again. I gave myself, and all I was slowly, slowly becoming, finally, after so many years of not knowing who I was at all.

I knew then, that up until now, I'd had no earthly idea how to be happy. Now I needed to learn. I gave myself to the sea too, knowing I loved myself deeply, as deeply as I loved my own child, knowing I was as responsible to myself as I was to him. And I gave my beloved grandmother who had not long ago faded into gaunt shadow and died. I gave it all, knowing I was whole and always would be, from here on out. I wiped my eyes and blew my nose and the sea pulled forever on.

My grandmother was why I had come here. She had sailed to Jersey alone when she was my age, just after the war had ended, unmarried and stubborn in her independence. I had wanted to share something of her spirit for a while. Her mother had worried about her, scolded her, tried to mould her, but Grandma had no time for that. She had always liked the sea, and to walk – laced-up boots, stout stick – at the kind of pace that even down a high street suggested wholesome air, pink cheeks, salt-tang. I couldn't match that, but I did find my way up to the very top of the cliff, walking slowly, coming to rest in the cold sunshine on the grass. It was here, or somewhere nearby, that she had met my grandfather, his shadow falling over her as she sat. They had exchanged a few polite words about the weather and the day. He, an older man, Polish and a divorcee – everything that would make her mother's eyes go wide. 'I have met the man I will marry,' she wrote home, soon after. And she had, and she did. My mother was born some years after.

I didn't expect to find love on the clifftop in some fateful echo, but I still held myself in readiness, braced, as if something might happen. I felt emptied of all sorrow. Would something come to fill me now? But all there was, was the call of gulls. The lichen curling yellow under the sun. The low white sun in the sky. And me, open and tender to myself and to the whole wide world.

I think maybe something did change that day. I think the silence woke up something inside me: the beginning of a new companionship with myself.

It didn't last, sustained, but then these things don't. Growth, becoming – it isn't a straight line: it's a spiral, round and round again, and it is painfully, painfully slow. So, first, next, I fall apart again, but then I get to come back. I'll bring new things with me, next time. I'll be better for it.

In the evening, I took myself for dinner. I was the only one in the restaurant and the waiters formed a line and sang an exuberant, tuneless happy birthday as they laid my pudding, fiery with sparklers, before my enchanted face.

★

Today there is sunshine. It coated my windows as it rose, liquid gold, meeting the condensation on my windows and setting it, crystalline. It looked like I should be able to scrape it off with a fingernail and put it in my mouth.

I dress and weave through the light to school and then to the community centre, and play songs from

Max Richter's recomposition of Vivaldi's *Four Seasons* on my headphones because the leaves are turning and I want to mark it. I will never tire of it for as long as I live: the season and music both.

I listen and I look at the day and – there, as I take my seat – the footsteps of a woman walking her dog past the window begin to match the rhythm of the repetitive pull of strings in my ears. I watch, and her dog's wagging tail synchronises, joining the beat.

My gaze shifts. A pause in the arrangement followed by a considered, swelling note coincides with a man bracing to leave his armchair opposite, veins thick on his hands, and a nose-scratch behind him catches the staccato note that follows. I watch a coat shrugged off in perfect 3/4 time. A slow cello joins and I watch an elderly woman raise knife and fork with each glide of the bow: a fragile, hesitant conductor. The leaf-fall responds outside, rolling into flurries of accelerando, the trees in the bright wind playing the air with their whole, wild bodies.

Thank goodness for the days when my tight, egotistical hold on a hoarded reality slips and I can see it all for what it is again: that nothing and no one is separate; that a playfulness fills the gaps between us; that this is all one conversation; one big song and dance. The roll of the seasons catches us up and spins us, dares us. So much around says 'I see you!' in its own way and challenges us to engage, to talk back, to play.

When you start to pay attention, so much aligns, knits, influences, that it becomes impossible not to believe that life must have some underlying melody, some inbuilt rhythm to which we're all secretly attuned, or could choose to join, if we relaxed long enough to feel it. It is tugging at us, all the time.

With my headphones on, I hear no words and so the people opening their mouths to talk in my view take on new sounds of high, tremulous strings, or deep rumbling bass. All are unknowingly turned into birds in an instant. A woman with a pink chin like a perfect circle says something to her companion and the quick stutter of violin fills the air, transforming her into a robin at dawn. Another stands and distractedly moves her gloves through her bare hands, fingers tapping against the leather: a clarinet joining the sound. A man raises his buttered toast with a crescendo and pauses, mid-air, to interject with a word, once, twice. Rise and pause and lower again, then rise and pause again, and I cannot help but lean forward to wait for the satisfaction of his eventual bite that lands, at last, with a convenient burst of the refrain.

The music builds. A woman with large, hoop earrings taps on a laptop, animato, and the quickening in my ears chases her fingers, faster, faster. I hold my breath. There is nothing but this, nothing but this perfect, mischievous orchestration of everything, and nobody knows, and nobody sees, so caught up in the seriousness of themselves and their day. I let it swell in my heart and my ears, until, until, it ends with a flourish, and the day waits to see what I'll do next.

The room is suddenly still, for a near-imperceptible moment, before moving to life again, and I have to sit on my hands to stop from bursting into impulsive, rapturous applause.

★

THEN

I had fallen in love. I hadn't meant to.

Mark was tall and charming and intense, his teeth bright when he smiled, his eyes creasing into irresistible folds when he looked at me, which he did, often, for just a little longer than anyone else ever had. We met for coffee and he touched the back of my neck, gently, just for a moment, as I stood on the high kerb to try and meet his eyes, and I was lost.

I was in the middle of a run of months of better energy, with not so many days spent in recovery when I pushed myself. I was well enough to be able to wander occasionally on the alternate weekends my son spent with his father, to roam further afield, to say yes again. My ex-husband had moved on, with a new girlfriend in tow, and so it was easier to let go of guilt there. My guilt lay with Mark and with his life. 'It's complicated,' he said, as men tend to say. I hadn't learned how often they say that, not yet. He wouldn't be the last man to say that to me or the one to wake in me what it meant.

We'd followed each other on Twitter and, somehow, I had become his confidant, comforter. I had caught a train to London to meet him, to look at art and to pretend to be sophisticated and stylish and to know about the world. He met me, grinning under his soft leather cap, long-legged like a puppy, his voice lilting close to my ear against the traffic noise. Oh, how I wanted him, all silence and peace in me burnt up like a match strike.

We played a hungry back-and-forth game for a while, of resistance and relenting, of gifts and promises, not seeing each other at all for months when I tried to put him from my mind and failed, until all will had crumbled and life began to revolve entirely around 'next time' – weekends of fevered bliss in his spacious, dark apartment, my body becoming something new with each hour together. Pleasure opened to me, surprised me, frightened me. In our weeks apart, I began to explore it tentatively, eagerly, on my own. I wanted to understand it, amazed to realise that my complex body could hold all this too.

One day I looked up and a year had gone by and I loved him more than I thought was possible. His voice, his laugh, the way he crossed his legs and frowned as he thought. 'This is what it's supposed to feel like, then,' I'd think, in the quiet of our shared nights as he slept next to me. I couldn't pull my eyes away from him. 'Ah, I see.' Later, I'd say the same thing about heartbreak.

My weekends there, I'd sit cross-legged on a dining chair, knitting, and watch him cook. He would sing as he did, his shoulders always a little hunched as if mid-shrug. I liked to watch his hands. He was a father to three wonderful, older boys – bright and loud, all limbs and moods. He shared equal custody with their mother who he hadn't divorced. He owned and ran a busy veterinary practice and came home smelling of dog, his hands rough, clever. He lived a lifestyle that I'd never even seen before, let alone shared in – luxurious, full of easy, confident entitlement. Things and choices that had always seemed alien to me, belonging to a different world, he just took them and helped me to take them too, knowing them his right, believing them my right too. Yes, there was dazzle in that, like someone turning a crystal in the light. I didn't want or need material things, but, oh, I wanted this *confidence*. He made adulthood feel powerful.

We'd drive to stylish restaurants and I'd watch the miles speed past as the sun set and be sure that this is what flying felt like: just like this. We went on holidays by the sea and found long, flat beaches to lose ourselves in, grinning behind our cameras as we took photos of each other under the wide sky. We played house. I stood next to him on a long pier in the sunshine, watching his hands grip the railing, feeling the strength and surety of him next to me and was certain I had found my home and my future.

To look back at those years is to think of a bright dream. I remember climbing a fence and bluebells, bluebells as far as I could see. I remember lying with him under canvas and the rain pummelling my senses, and laughing and laughing, happiness made beautifully, suddenly real, as if I'd been handed it like a new child.

★

Today was supposed to be warm. Everyone's been talking about it. An Indian Summer, they said, twenty-two degrees promised, and so I dressed obligingly. And it has been warm, it has. I have looked around and seen sleeves rolled up and more bare leg than I've seen in a month, and yet I've shivered through it, persistently, stubbornly. I have shivered through it all.

There is often a feeling of being separate from this existence. My bubble of chill made it tangible today: them in their bright ease, me, bundled, as if unable to bear their world. I have been a ridiculous extraterrestrial, shuddering, looking in slow-blinked, can't-take-it-in pauses at the leaves beginning to heap in the gutters.

When will I learn how to live here? Another decade? Another three? I sit and watch orange leaves fall past my window; one, then another, steady, pirouetting. As if to mock me, my body, suddenly panicked, unleashes a torrent of sweating, disproportionate, embarrassed, like a dog barking too loudly. It tries to catch up to the warmth of the day and pretend it is human. It does a good impression of it and I sit and let it, until it reverts to its usual chill again.

But, later, when I am outside, unarmed, I see that it isn't just me that is strange today. The light is flat and sharp, its dimensions compressed. The leaves in the gutters I had gawped at earlier seem to glow with a light that shouldn't be there. I can't work out where the light is coming from, to make them glow like that. The sun skulks low, the shadows long. I am thrown from light to shadowy dark every few feet in disorientating contrast. And yet even in the shadows, the leaves continue to glow with light from that hidden sun, and I think, I am not the only one detached from something normal today. I am not the only one unfitting.

There are roses in the school kitchen window, but they are dead and wrinkled; heads dipped on broken necks. A girl skips ahead of me in a pale blue sundress, both straps slipped, and her bare shoulders look blue too, mottled. I am struck, suddenly, that it is not as warm as we all think it is today; not as alive as we've convinced ourselves either. Maybe I'm not the wrong one after all. I have this awful feeling that we've propped up summer's corpse to take tea with. None of it seems quite right today. Not just me – I never feel quite right – but all of it. I'm afraid that we're holding onto something that isn't here any more.

A parcel arrives from Denmark that smells, overwhelmingly, of home, safety, sleep. I weep into it. Ah, perhaps that is the problem after all. How I miss him.

Fraser flew over two weeks ago for a brief weekend to celebrate his birthday with us – his fiftieth. So soon after last time, it felt as though we'd cheated some system. It felt like more than I deserved, but I took it.

Afterwards, I tried not to erase the markers of him that remained around the house, knowing I was simply prolonging the inevitable but stubbornly resisting it all the same. I kept his half-drunk glass of water by the bed. When washing dishes, I paused and put his coffee mug back on the counter to sit unwashed another day. I pushed my nose into his t-shirt in the washing basket and left that for the next wash too. Sometimes now, I spray a little of his cologne in the air and step into it like an embrace, just for a moment, just until it fades. Sometimes I wonder what on earth I have done to myself in finally opening to try again like this only for it to be in a form that must remain so sporadic and fleeting.

I tell myself perhaps it's safer for me like this, to be reminded so starkly that nothing lasts. I can't take it for granted this way. I can better learn to gather in and let go again, or better try to, at least.

I am shivering again. I think I'm getting another cold. I wonder if I'll manage to suffer through it calmly and dispassionately and conclude that I probably will not.

★

THEN

Not long after Mark and I met, I had begun to lose consciousness at strange moments. In the shower and after eating, especially. I'd feel my tongue thicken and blackness begin to pour in at the edges, my heart getting faster and faster until everything lost its clarity. I'd have to lie down there and then, wherever I was, feeling the thump thump thump. 'I'm so sorry,' I'd say, 'I'm not feeling well.'

At Mark's, I'd sleep, embarrassed, ashamed to have spoiled the day. At home, I'd sit my son next to me in bed and play nature programmes while I recovered. He was long used to a mother who got tired and woozy and I smiled through it, as I always did, so he wouldn't be afraid. I wondered what it meant and assumed it probably meant nothing, just like everything else my body did. Pain had crept back too: a heavy, intense pressure in my legs, especially at night or after walking, leaving me sleepless, weary. I'd take a pill and try to push it from my mind.

I put off going to the doctor's until I couldn't any more, until it began to get dangerous. It would sometimes take a while for my speech to return properly after a fainting attack, my limbs buzzing with electricity. Echocardiograms and monitoring showed my heart was healthy but that I was experiencing occasional episodes of sudden, severe tachycardia. They said it was nothing to worry about. The doctors talked about panic attacks, about anxiety. 'No, no that's not what's happening,' I'd say. 'I'm so happy! This is the happiest I've ever been!' I woke up once on a tube platform, a circle of faces around me. 'We're getting you some help,' they said, but I slurred, 'No, no, I'm fine,' and stumbled onto the train before they could do anything else. I just wanted to get home.

I tried to put it from my mind. There was so much good to focus on and I breathed it in and out, slow and steady. And a new life was growing, maybe, if I was patient. Something safe and brave and full of love. It would all be OK.

★

The thermometer says 40.1 degrees and the world has begun to warp. It is only a cold only a cold only a cold. I say it like a runaway train. My body doesn't understand appropriate reactions to colds or to trains or anything else. My fingers have gone numb at the tips. I press them to things, trying to programme myself right again, my skin buzzing. Wrong. Wrong.

I have been shaking violently. A trip to the toilet resulted in a slumped faint on the bathroom floor and my tongue feels thick in my mouth now. My face feels strange, like not all of it is mine. There is a pain in my pelvis, hot and loud. None of this is unusual. I brought myself round quietly, my son downstairs and unaware, as I have done many times before. I sit looking at the unlit, black rectangle of my phone, back in bed now, wondering whether to call somebody. I can't remember when I last did that and I am reluctant to now because I know it is all probably meaningless. I have learnt after many false alarms that although my body's messages to me are real and disabling, they're often misleading and not a sign of danger: clanging physical reactions, all sound and fury signifying only that my body is struggling, in its strange, unfathomable way. This is not how bodies are supposed to work.

A storm on the stairs and my son appears. He wraps his arms around me and presses his head to mine. I try to make words come out but all I can think of is how hot he feels against me. God, how can anything be so hot? Maybe it is him who is sick, not me. Maybe

I've got even that wrong? I can say nothing but small things.

'Are you feeling OK?' I ask him, backwards.

'I'm fine. You have a sleep, Mummy,' he says, and goes back downstairs, but I can't sleep.

Memory of humiliation sits stifling around me in the hot room. The times I made everyone worry for nothing. The invasion of tests, driven by my body's odd behaviour, so many tests, that usually led nowhere – too many to count. Gowns that didn't do up at the back. Cold faces, cold questions, the waiting and waiting and the wondering each time only to be told it was nothing to be overly concerned about after all. Ride it out. Ride it out. Now I am afraid of medical attention and more judgement, of wasting others' time. It has created a phobia in me so strong that I have lost the ability to see a doctor now without silent, freezing distress and I avoid going much at all. But I am also afraid of getting sick with something else and none of us realising until damage is done, because that is the cruellest thing about all of this: that I know I can't discount the alarm bells entirely.

One day, hidden amongst the noise, there might be a message that could save my life. For the sake of the people that love me, I can't just ignore everything, always, cheerfully cutting my body off from all attention or medical care. And so, still, part of me wonders with each new extremity: am I doing the

right thing? Should I call someone? Is this different?
Is it dangerous, this time?

'I don't know what to do,' I say, rocking, my head in
my hands. No wonder I don't know what to believe
on days like this. No wonder I doubt. This is the result
of years of being ill, then not ill, but always ill again, all
the time no one convinced I was really ill at all – not
even me. This is the trauma. This is what makes me
still feel, often, so profoundly unsafe because I can't
escape my own body and I can't trust it.

I have avoided saying whether I think the different
doctors I've seen were right or wrong about me
because as the years go on, it matters less and less.
Whatever they think, I must still live, somehow. I must
live through days like this.

I know now, as well as I can ever know anything,
that my body just doesn't work the way it should. But
I know too that my mind is complicated. It suffers
and gets confused and led astray; it affects my body in
strange and unexpected ways. It draws on the safety
or lack of it in my environment, on my thoughts, on
my experiences. It does this because I am a human
being. There is no shame in that for me now. I know
I am no different in that than anyone else around me.

Now, this line we draw above the neck seems
laughable. As if our head and body live entirely
different lives, with some borderline drawn clear
between mental and physical health; identity, activity

and ownership ring-fenced, assigned the appropriate identity and paperwork. As if that could be true, or helpful. It's as meaningless as the idea of any sovereign land. It's all just more 'them and us'.

Knowing all this, I sit and watch the phone, trying to stay in my skin. There is no reconciling it. I can never know for certain whether I'm making the right choices. I can only try to steer my mind towards calm, towards reason and wise action and forgive myself, over and over, when I get it wrong. To recognise that my mind and my body aren't my fault, but they are my responsibility.

I gather the feeling in my hands like clay. I draw in the hope, lost and new, the doubt, the fierce terror, the unfailing, undrainable joy that I can't let go of, that I am made of despite everything, and I hold it and pat it softly with my hands. The why of it doesn't matter. I must simply care for myself through all of it, so I do.

I run a hand down my arm and whisper, 'I will take care of you,' and my body shifts from abuser and back to the wild, frightened animal it always was, to a child, to my child and my greatest gift. I forgive it anew, as I always would my boy.

'Always, always. I promise. You are safe here. Look, you are safe. I will always take care of you. I am glad of you, fragile one. I am glad of you, but you don't have to do this alone.'

I take a deep breath, and I dial.

★

THEN

We didn't see Mark's friends or family much, if at all – I was told that was complicated too – but I didn't mind it. I loved our solitary weekends, many spent with our collected boys in a perfect, rowdy racket.

I would seize at the chance to hang their clothes to dry. It felt like being allowed downstairs at a grown-up party. Their bigger shirts and shorts, socks and hoodies, would tumble easily into my arms, affectionate and indulgent, and I, wide-eyed, intoxicated, would lead them to their places on the clothes dryer, smitten with their familiarity yet drawn to the otherness of their maturity. They smelled rich and confident, of something in charge and good to trust. Occasionally, I would offer a few of my own or my son's things into the mix, and they'd languish between them, enjoying their temporary identity as one of them.

I'd look at the six of us together and think 'family' like a new question, slowly building the courage I knew it would take to move to be with him one day, to make a change, to seize this future and take my place at his side until all our clothes smelt like theirs. The conflict it might spark terrified me but, oh, I wanted this new life. It was all I wanted, until his estranged wife came across me in the supermarket one afternoon. She saw me, horror in her face, her back arching like a cat, and hissed that they weren't mine, weren't mine to have, not even Mark. '*My* family,' she spat, she sobbed, and I watched the word die, seeing her pain.

He listened to that story as I told him later, swallowing, unchallenging, as I shook with distress. I had tried to talk to him about our future, over weeks, months, trying to find the right moment, the right words. 'Are you ready? Ready for us to think about . . . ready to plan for more?' and the answer was always, no, no.

I laughed, weeping, at what I saw as my stupidity afterwards, when he broke it off. I'd done exactly what I'd said I wouldn't do and imagined a better future than this one, for me and my boy, and thinking it still lay in the power of another and far away, I had run towards it. I thought he'd be the one to help us find our way; that we'd make it together; that he'd help me be brave, and that maybe I'd help him be brave too. I thought he loved me, and perhaps he did for a little while, until one day he didn't, or not enough in any case.

His mother, a retired GP, had said, 'You need to watch women with illnesses like hers. They're usually after something. They want to be looked after.' I had laughed hollowly at that, fiery in my independence, knowing she'd got it all wrong. It wasn't anything as insidious as care that I wanted, no, it was something far more unlikely: boring, simple happiness with this man that I adored. A chance to prove myself, yes, maybe, but mostly just to live, bold and confident; to live a life I thought might fit me. To be brave and free. To belong at last. To be loved, that's all, as much as I loved him.

'I'm just not ready,' he told me when he ended it. 'I already have so much responsibility here. I need some time, to work out who I am and what I want, to focus on what matters to me.' The drawing of that line hung in the air between us and I watched it crack and burn up every bit of safety and assurance I had imagined, all over again.

I waited, for a long while, hoping, denying, until I found out he'd moved back in with his wife and not told me. I stopped waiting then.

I was lost for a while.

I tried to make sense of it, sitting in the ash of the home I had imagined. I told myself that nice things weren't meant for me. I told myself that this was my punishment for being greedy and for causing so much hurt. I tried to move on with my life, but the new grief was a boulder, wide and weighty, and I felt it every day. There were moments when I had to sit on the floor with the mass of it, my legs giving way, nothing making sense but the ground. I had never known a sensation like this loss, every cell of my body swelling to try and hold it. And I missed him. I missed him so much, and the boys – the thought of his boys was like a bullet wound. There were days when I thought it would split me. 'What if I can't bear it?' I'd say to the empty air, heaving, so angry I wanted to pull the clean room down around me until it looked like the ruin I felt. 'What then?' But I did bear it, of course, because somehow you do, and time passed, and life went on. I know I felt outrage at that too at times.

Now I understand there was no shame in wanting him. There was nothing weak in it. There is nothing wrong with wanting to share a life, and to share it well. That will always be a precious gift to offer. It wasn't my fault that he didn't, couldn't, want it back. It wasn't his fault either. He wasn't ready: he'd told the truth there, and sometimes truth hurts.

This is why my joy now is brave. I need you to know that. I know what it means to try and to see something fail, and I know it can happen over and over.

This is why I'm still afraid, so often. Because I know how these things can go.

★

I lie flat on my bed. My legs thrum and pound somewhere on their usual horizon. A bright spot in my back pulls and aches. The cat comes to sit next to me and makes small sounds by my ear; a huff–puff of breath, impatient. I can hear the wet, busy sounds of his tongue. With the sounds, time makes sense again and I align to it, like two pendulums swinging in sync. I raise a wrist to my nose and smell the perfume there too, to find a similar beat. Ah yes. Three days have passed since I called the doctor. My fever turned out to be an infection after all. I am woozy on antibiotics and trying to heal again.

I forget that healing feels like loss. For a long time, I thought suffering was something you outgrew, outpaced, by being happy and working hard. I think part of me still thought I might be able to leave it behind now that I have found safe love, written out my story, found my voice, built a life of good habits. Perhaps still, deep down, I held hope that one day I would find the combination of thoughts and choices that loosened pain and fear and illness so powerfully, it could do nothing but leave me entirely, forever, even though I know that what I'm describing could only mean death.

Pain may not feel pleasant or convenient, but at least it means I'm still here. Today, the pulse to my legs, my back, my head, feels extraordinary. All these years and on those nerves buzz and clamour, tirelessly, telling me their stories. They are as eager to live as I am. There comes with it, suddenly, a profound gratitude that they haven't given up on me.

I believe now that within pain, within everything, there might be a chance for me to discover *more* about what it means to be alive, not less. Pain might be a doorway, not a fist. It's the fear that makes it worse – it's the fear that makes it unbearable – so maybe if I can tackle the fear, today and every day, one day suffering will simply become another moment of curiosity to experience and explore.

It feels like my last and biggest confession, that I am still so often afraid. I am afraid of my delinquent body. I am afraid that a hand will come down on my fragile, careful life. I am afraid that the numbers don't add up and that soon there will be a reckoning. I am afraid of worse. I am even afraid of better, because then I will have more to lose. So many days, I sit and rot in fear's clench and berate myself for being back there, but then healing is never linear. Healing contains stinking pockets that you can fall into at any time. It doesn't have to be a smooth upward trajectory from here on in and no progress is ever lost because there's nowhere to arrive at. What matters, simply, is that you make a home, a place of peace to come back to and rest in when you need to, whenever you can. The more you do it, the easier it gets.

That is the beauty of mind. I was taught to be afraid of that too, once, but now I know it is my greatest power, my greatest strength. Now I know, when I fall into that fearful place, to nod and peel open my fear like overripe fruit, piecing through the mess of it. I find the hard stone in each and every terror is the same: I am afraid that I will be made to feel something I can't handle. That I'll split open like bad fruit myself; I'll tear right down the middle and my mind will crack and I will be gone. A nonsense. Have I ever before? Have I not lived through every fear and held?

Now, I chase each worst fear right to the end, playing out every worst case scenario and when I do that, I know that each story ends with 'and then I adapt, and keep going, and in time, I am OK again,' and I remember that I don't need to be afraid of anything, because my ability to bend and grow is limitless.

All that's left is to soothe myself until the fear passes. Safety lies with me, in my words, in my marvellous, malleable mind, in the small actions of my day.

I finish knitting the sock that has lain beside me on my bed and turn my thoughts to its partner. When I feel well enough, I make my way down the stairs on my bottom and call to my boy. He makes me a cup of tea. Together, we gather in the washing from the cold, yellow garden, and watch a gull in the sky, the low sun catching its underbelly. I close my eyes and say a prayer to no one, in thanks, in hope. I put my hand to my heart and feel the hard flutter there, like I've swallowed the bird from the air, and I know I will never, ever be undone, not entirely. I have a place of calm to come back to now, however hard life gets, and no one can pull it down.

Healing is a way of life, a lived intention, a way of behaving. I will never not need it and never get to leave it behind. It runs right the way through who I am now.

I can let myself be a new being every day, if I need to. How hard it is. How confusing and tiring, but possible, possible.

★

THEN

I want to say that the stillness was waiting for me, after Mark, but nothing waits for us, not really. It's in waiting in our own fixed place, waiting for whatever it is to find us, that we waste so much time. There is only ever what we hunt out and find, stepping forward across a gap to invite it back inside, knowing that sometimes it will say no, or not yet, but that we must ask anyway. I did that. I stepped back into that still place I had found on the clifftop in Jersey two years before, and I asked, 'Will you have me back?' and it said yes.

I began to walk, often and alone, in a blue hat I knitted myself, in purple wellies that I wore until the rubber rotted itself thin. I didn't go far and not for long, tiring quickly as I always had, but I still felt like the whole world was mine. Slowly, I healed, watching lapwings tumble over the marshlands near my house, tucked between the industrial estates and the big graveyard. I made a second home in the squat, dirty bird hide by the biggest lake and I went every day, for a little while at least. I climbed trees and lay in the branches. I learned the calls of teal, tufted ducks, grebe, water rail, snipe, cormorant. I watched them until each were as familiar as old hands.

★

A woman has been sat across from me for an hour, her old, pink trainers flat on the floor of the community centre. It is the first time I've been here in over a fortnight but I am doing a little better so I came. Her large body is unmoving in the sofa cushions. She has looked around once or twice, hands motionless, but mostly her gaze has rested low, on nothing in particular, or, eyes closing, she has dozed while her mouth fell a little open.

She could be meditating, or drugged, or depressed, or at peace and resting in the day. She could be hiding, avoiding, or waiting. I cannot tell. One arm curls loosely around a red leather bag. Her hair is pulled back simply.

Whoever she is, whyever she is here, I am struck with a simple gratitude that there is a space for people to rest here, companionably, unchallenged. We move around her, or sit still ourselves, and she is safe and not alone.

It isn't just rest we need: it's safe rest. It's only in safety that we can heal, and we make that safety for each other.

I will keep vigil, friend. I will keep vigil while you stop too.

★

THEN

My serious boy grew and laughed and scrunched up his face at things he didn't like, and he loved me and his dad and his time with each of us, without question, with every inch of his small, wriggling body. He loved superheroes and pirates and wham-bam battles and dancing and jokes and storytime, demanding that I read *Fox in Socks* by Dr Seuss faster and faster, grinning as I sped through tongue twisters until I'd fall down on his pillow, defeated, so he could bury his jubilant face in my chest. He was suspicious of food and new things and clothes that weren't soft. Although he still struggled with language he was growing sociable and confident. 'He probably just needs time,' his health visitor had said, and I knew she was right.

When he had started school, the money had run out. In the three years we'd lived on our own, I had struggled over and over to find a way to keep us solvent.

Childcare was an impossible, complex expense, and so, month by month, I had stayed at home to care for him, making do with welfare and less, using what free nursery hours we were offered to study a funded, long-distance arts course, hoping that maybe I could train to be a teacher one day. But on his fifth birthday, my Income Support was stopped – new rules for single parents, they said. The only option was to sign on as a jobseeker.

Unskilled and unqualified meant my choices lay back in care work or cleaning, neither of which my body would be able to cope with for long, but I didn't want to be signed off sick again. There must be something I could do that wouldn't mean too much time on my feet; I was sure of it. My walks and my time on the marshes had nurtured a new strength in me in recent months and I had always loved to work. I knew I had a lot to give again. I was ready.

I hunted and hunted for part-time office work that I could fit around school hours, but it didn't seem to exist, not here. Librarian positions in schools appeared to be a thing of the past and rare school support-work positions were fiercely competed for. I expanded the search area over a wider and wider area and felt sick just thinking of the hours on buses. I thought again about university, but there was no financial support for part-time students, and full-time study was still beyond me. The amount I'd have to borrow in either case was terrifying; I didn't even know if I could. The nearest university was two train rides away. My son was still in therapy for his disordered speech, still settling into school, and he needed me at home. He was the most enduring, important thing in my life. I wanted to be a smiling face at the gate and a hand to hold on the way home, just for a little while longer, until he was surer of himself. The thought of losing more time together after losing everything else felt devastating.

I tried to talk to my caseworker at the Jobcentre, but she looked at me under the straight line of her fringe, her eyes unmoved by my talk of our needs, of my ambition, of art and teaching. She said that making do was the best someone in my situation could hope for and that it was time to let go of unrealistic dreams. It was time to be practical. If I didn't commit to getting a job, I'd be sanctioned and lose my benefits, did I understand that? No, there were no training schemes suitable for me. Did I know how to write a CV? There was a workshop for that. Yes, yes, I knew how to do that. She signed me up anyway.

At first, I went through the motions, scouring the jobs websites each day in hope something suitable would come up, but an anger in me grew. This time, rather than succumbing to the powerlessness they said was my place, some old fire in me said 'no.'

It was time to be practical, she'd said, and she was right, but I was going to choose how.

★

It's blowing a gale here. It's shaking the buddleia that grows out from the narrow gap beside next door's garage, bricks bulging around its thickening trunk. I have stayed home from my usual hour at the community centre with a reflushing of fever and pain to read my book.

'Oooh, oooh.' The wind is breathless in the chimney, the door knocker pat-pats itself. I stop to bury my face in the downy mound of my cat's tummy, dangerous, irresistible. He stretches his hind legs out and along the sofa now, straight and bandy like a Cossack in fur trousers.

I am reading *The Telling*, by Ursula K. Le Guin. I have read very little else but her books this year, one after another. Nothing else will do. I turn the pages, sinking into it, lulled, until I am brought to an abrupt stop. I have found an interesting idea, here on the page, like a rich, sweet note, sung in harmony with my own. My ears prick up with it, my heart quickens with belonging. One of *those* kinds of ideas. I read it again. Then again.

Here is what she tells. Natural things – animals, birds, rivers, plants – they all have an instinct, a natural way of being that guides them from birth to death.

They need no interference, only for their own nature to be allowed to exist in the right environment. Beyond that, all will flow.

But us humans, we are empty. Our nature is chaotic and flawed. Without carers and caretakers, we will not learn how to exist in our world. We will not know how to stay safe or how to thrive. Without help from the start and on through our lives, without parents and teachers and communities, we will die. Because of that, we are what we're taught. We become what we're told. The telling comes through what we hear, what we read, what we are exposed to, and where we choose to focus our time. It shapes us, our actions, our being, our choices. And we can be told good ways of being in the world, good ways to use and treat our bodies, our power, our thoughts, energies, desires, identities – all of them – and we can be taught bad ways. We can be taught ways that heal and grow ourselves and our communities and families along with us, or we can be taught harmful ways that poison, damage, divide, us and others too.

It's all in the telling: in the stories we learn and believe and pass on through our words and behaviours.

It is a devastating and thrilling idea. I sit back and swallow it as I listen to the 'oooh, oooh' of the chimney, and the pat-pat of door knocker, and the bang of the back gate, warped beyond locking.

Some days I wonder what all this listening and looking is for, but the more I do it, the more I start to see the stories I've been told for what they are. I see how they've shaped me; I notice their footprint in my reactions, my thoughts. By stopping to listen, to look, I think maybe I leave a space in which I might learn new, truer, more helpful stories. I acknowledge that the world itself might be able to teach me what I need to know next, maybe even better than people can.

I think these thoughts and the cat stands and stretches, does two turns on the spot like a spell and settles down again into a tight ball, his tongue clicking twice, contentedly.

★

THEN

I joined a business start-up course designed to get people out of unemployment and sat around the long table, defiant, determined, in a smart skirt and proper shoes. When it came to my turn to share my idea, I looked the advisor straight in the eye and said I was going to write persuasive, passionate words for money; words that cut straight to the heart of things. 'Words that will make people feel something, then act,' I said. Words on documents, websites, leaflets, personal statements, elevator pitches: I could turn anything into something that people would want to read and respond to. And everyone else in this room wanting to launch a business? I could help them sell it.

Within a month, the advisor at the Chamber of Commerce had hired me himself. Alongside, he helped me compile a business plan, a cashflow, and a marketing strategy. Two more people from our start-up group offered work and promised more. I made myself a website. I registered as self-employed and, with a new leap and a deep breath, stopped signing on. I read every book on marketing and copywriting that had ever been written and I blagged my trembling heart out. I wrote beautiful, powerful words. I wrote daring pitches. I contacted charities and marketing agencies, and even travelled to meet people face-to-face when I could, smiling and confident – a professional in disguise. I did as I'd always done: I hid my fatigue, my doubt, collapsing only afterwards, and slowly, slowly, my business and reputation started to grow. Clients sent me heartfelt thank yous. I sent off invoices and felt a flush as the money hit my bank account. Not a lot, but enough, *enough*. To my great surprise, I discovered I was good at this, after all.

I'd walk the marshes between contracts and wonder if I was on the right track. I didn't think I was, not yet – it felt like a role I was acting, other people's words in my mouth and not who I was – but it was a start and that would do. I'd got the Jobcentre off my back and put food on the table. Potential spread from my feet like tributaries and I saw I could follow one path, or another, and that it didn't really matter which because I could always change things on the way.

'Not now,' I'd say to the train in my chest when it galloped me back into unconsciousness, my bottom muddy on the path where I'd slumped, to the pain in my legs that had begun to get louder and louder again. 'Not now.'

★

It is raining. I am in bed again and the grey sky is smudging into the grey-painted house opposite, colour running off everything like cheap hair dye.

White-faced, my eyes blue plums of fatigue, I have let myself be pulled back and down. There is nothing to push against again today, nothing to fight. To fight, there needs to be something to resist against and in this slow, liquid sink there is none of that.

Propped up on pillows to stop me from tipping and falling, I spend the day as I spend many. Not thinking; writing, when I can.

Books have been pulled around me, like great, aligned stones, with me their still centre. My notebook and my pen lie by my side. To watch me, you would see only a few words written at a time. When I stop being able to lift my arm to write, I read a little, or lie back, eyes closed, and let my mind play. I watch the wet world outside and imagine golden fish twisting in shoals around the lampposts; the wheelie bins morphing into ponderous hermit crabs, trailing across sandy pavements; the sudden rush of a car a wide, red whale. You can dream your way through ideas, through pain, I have learned. You don't have to control it all: if there is no control left, it's OK. Your mind will make great leaps, jumping gaps between things to find out what's on the other side. You can let thought swim through you, and you can write it out, in ebbs and flows. Slow, slow.

When there is no energy or focused thought, you must write deep from your body. It's all that's left of you. You must do it in steady, gentle heaves, like an animal breathing. You must see your chance and move, quick and wild, scuttling to the light or the shadow, then hide, hide, rest, rest.

And so, today, I write with my body. I write with my undignified, clamouring body. I write with cold fingers unsteady around my pen. My arm shifts and drives like a slow, slow piston, pulling the words from me a handful at a time, nudging them out. They gather in my stomach as I rest. I gather it all in the middle, and then I write with my arched back, curved forward and hollow and taut, like a ready bow, just for a moment, till I'm spent. I wait for it to build again, for a silent tide of words to swell. A sentence, two – it's rarely much more – and the rain keeps falling in silent torrents around me.

I write with my frozen feet and my red, swollen toes. I stop. I write with my tight mouth and my hard frown and the cheap, untidy clothes I pulled on this morning. I stop again. I write with the hard knot of my aching womb and the hidden whiteness of my thighs, with the stubble of my armpits that I had no energy to shave, and the tangle of my hair. Stop. Write. Stop. Write. Sometimes there is serenity in it. Often there is love, because love will always quicken your heart and you can channel it down into your pen, and so I have learned to pounce on love, for fuel, for succour. Fury works too, my insides pushing some mass of me out, panicked and angry; like a heartbroken woman emptying a house. I prefer to fall in love, if I can, but with no other energy left, I will take what I can.

Either way, I must simply lay one sentence down, then rest, and then lay down another. It often hurts to do it. I take comfort in the fact that although other writers will get to write more quickly or with more dignity, when all else is taken away, all they're left with is laying down one sentence after another too and it is probably just as painful for them, in different ways.

Today I write at a snail's pace, without show, but word by word, it still grows and that is the greatest peace of all. I used to tell myself I would never be able to write a book, that it was another unachievable dream I'd have to let go of, but look, I almost have.

My heart is a jackrabbit. I rest, I sleep. I wake and pull my notebook close again and write more words in a shaking hand a little at a time. I am a being of movement and growth, determined, unstoppable and the earth comes up to meet me. Through the floor, through the spaces in the empty rooms that wait for my son to come home, up through the bed.

I am not separate. With just a little reach, I become an extension of the sway of conifer in the wind and the pace of the man with hunched shoulders who walks his small, grey dog past my window, hidden in his hood. I become his shuffling feet and his blank stare. I become the neighbour backing her car out of a tight space, who I know twists her wedding ring and bites her hair. My dark eyes are black beetles and the tightness in me is the middle of a mountain. I nod and the pigeons on the rooftops nod; I breathe in slow and deep and the clouds move. I let my pen move across the page like a heartbeat, keeping it all alive. I become its will, its desire and its fear and I know that, in that, I have a purpose and always will do now, however slow I go and however many times I fail.

I know others don't see it in me, but I don't need them to any more. I suspect that this is why they chop down trees, because they mistake stillness for passivity, stupidity. I am not afraid. Not afraid to lose, or to be less. I am just so glad to be here.

Besides: the audacity of it, of writing anything at all. Hidden deep in a society where I am supposed to be a machine that only works, consumes, pretends, and then begs for more, I rest and I pull darkness and beauty, pure truth and make-believe right out of the air.

No one can stop me.

★

THEN

The doctor said that my tachycardia would improve if I worked on my fitness levels, so I did that next. I worked and I swam and swam and stretched and built muscle and even ran a little, some days, all the way down the hidden path past the marshes, reaching my fingers to brush the leaves on the low trees, feeling as free as a swallow. I felt my body grow toned and strong. I liked that, pausing at the mirror to follow the new hollows and shapes of me, stretching and moving in my yoga classes to feel my body holding me firm. I saw men's gaze catch me as I walked about my life. I joined a dating website and went on a date, then another one, and smiled over bourbon and ice.

But even at my fittest, I still fainted on the floor of my living room when I got home from my runs, and at the swimming pool after each swim, hidden in the bottom of a cubicle, instructors knocking on the door. I began to suspect this wasn't going to magically go away. I was everything they had ever told me to be: active, happy, responsible, ambitious, confident, fit, and still my body didn't work the way it was supposed to. I began to laugh at that, at this grand lie I had been told my whole life. I'd laugh as I picked myself up off the floor yet again, mouth thick, pain thrumming and thrumming. What on earth was I supposed to do now?

My response was to get a tattoo that ran the length of my torso, from ribs to thigh – botanical peonies and roses and chrysanthemums, hiding bees, butterflies, a caterpillar, a snail. Each petal and stem was inked bold and slow, and as I watched it grow over two long sittings, I thought of stars stuck to a little girl's hospital bed. It was an act of reclamation. When I dressed again afterwards, you could see no sign of it. With it, I took back my body and made it my own again. I knew I was strong now. I knew I was sane, and no one was going to take that away from me again.

I was invited to give the keynote speech at the Chamber of Commerce AGM and fainted in front of the Mayor, our MP, representatives from the local council and thirty noted business owners, mid-speech. When I'd recovered, I stood back up and finished my talk. 'I have this disability, you see,' I said, flushing scarlet but defiant, owning it for the first time. 'I don't really understand it, but I'm living the best life I can anyway.'

They all stood and clapped. I knew I held more power in that moment than all of them.

★

I turn right instead of left and go the long way home despite the rain. After days of being stuck in bed, I woke with a sudden panic and a need to know that everything was still there, but the sky looks the same above me, the clouds keep on and the rain still falls, and I have to conclude that all endures as it ever did.

The footpath I head to cuts between the boundary of our estate and the marshes in one meandering line, dropped below the level of the main roads, weaving under them through dark tunnels, hidden unless you know it's there. An old railway line. An edge place: dirty and riotous. The trees are young and they grow where they please. In the green months, the borders heave out a hedgerow unique to places like this: the prim botanist's favourites all jumbled up with deeply urban life. It is a place of hooded dog walkers and cyclists and fly-tipping and graffiti and all manner of good, wild things. This is where I used to run, once.

Today all is withered, soaked, spent. I go slow. There isn't a soul here and so I let myself move my scooter wheels at a crawl, through the ivy ink and bramble brown, the thick mush of leaves. The only bright colour comes from carrier bags and spray paint. Birch trees cradle the path like boned fingers. It is a dead and hollow place and my love of it rushes back in a wave as the rain pelts down.

There is no washing clean of anything within it. There is just a kind of grim resistance to the air and to the lines and shapes of everything. Oh, we're still here, I feel it say, its laugh hollow around me. Oh, we're still here all right.

The rain had hit the thinning canopy and branching forks, deflecting, and now its rivulets join to form long, thin, snaking rivers down the trunks. As I creep, the trees weep from knothole eyes, blank, unblinking, impenetrable. I do not think they weep for us. Our contributions to this place are not favourable: a used condom threaded onto an erect twig, rubbery and milky and provocative; a peg on another from a forgotten washing line between the trees; a mass of soggy cardboard. The graffiti under the bridges speak of anger, not beauty. I make myself notice each thing.

The trees make my ceiling and I can see every lung line of them. I can see them try to breathe. My feet don't touch the ground, but I try to press my own roots down to find them, to find something to hold, to see, but there is nothing but glowering sky and branch. It grips me in its giant nest, and I want to say, I see it all, I love you, I am so very sorry.

When the blackbird comes into my path, I wonder, for a moment, if it will take to my shoulder right there and then, in undeserved forgiveness and benediction, so that we can continue onwards together, but a jogger passes and startles it before it can. My unexpectedly young face under my deep hood makes him miss a step and I beam at him like a mischievous gnome as he recovers himself. And in that moment, that is what I become, as much a part of this place as everything around me, and the patter and the sway of it says yes, you are ours. Like it or not, I know I am home.

At the end of the next tunnel ahead, I can see the silhouette of a man standing in the middle of the dark path, his back to me.

Two full shopping bags have been dropped at his feet. He stands, arms by his side, and gazes out; a strange sentinel over the neglected footpath. I half imagine he will call out as I approach, his features still hidden from me. A riddle to solve, perhaps, or a judgement to pass. But he doesn't turn until I am level with him, distracted as he is, lost in whatever holds his thoughts on the horizon. A rueful, half-embarrassed smile scuttles up his unremarkable face, as if running to tidy up and make itself respectable again.

'The weather isn't so nice today,' he says simply, and I affirm, smiling back with words I don't remember, simply a dripping-wet girl in a raincoat again.

I leave him in that dark, dry pausing place and press on, wondering if I have, perhaps, passed or failed some test after all.

★

THEN

I began to write again for pleasure then for the first time since my marriage ended, in private, thick journals, not showing them to anyone. Dangerous words – not words for sale, but words for me. Thoughts, feelings. Things I saw and things I felt. Secret things and true.

They felt horribly, wonderfully indulgent. I had been told to be useful, to make my skills pay in a way that was respectable and impressive, but these words did nothing but scream and laugh. I preferred them. I'd bunk off my contracts to write them, in the bird hide, in my bed, in cafés, on the stairs as my son watched television and played his loud games. These journals sit on my shelves now as a record of my life since – the last four years in observations and stories, changing, growing, full of long gaps between the dates when I wandered off track and then found my way back again. I always found my way back.

In them, I see the same thoughts turned over and over. I drew ideas to me and pushed them away. I wrote about the litter-strewn natural world around

357

me, the snails in my garden, the geese that flew in great arrows over the house, the people I passed in the street. I wrote about another kind but unavailable 'it's complicated' man, who I knew better than to want and who I wished I could quit. I wrote about my mother, and about my father who had just remarried again, who I'd grown close to and away from and close to again. I wrote about my new friend Jude. I wrote about the worsening days of illness and prised open my fatigue and pain and love and desire and purpose and all of it.

I was often frustrated and ashamed of myself, and yet reading the journals back now, I can see how much power they contained. Every time I turned over a moment, a thought, an idea, I began to make a choice. I began to move towards something. Little by little, through my mistakes and my corrections, I came ever closer to what I really wanted to say and how I wanted to live.

This time, when I finally became too ill to keep going again, when life brought me once again to a stop: this time, I was ready.

★

The dark October sky, the glide of the wheels underneath me and the zip of a full battery when all the day's previous movement had been a sluggish strain, and here it is again: bliss.

I am moving between my house and Jude's on my scooter, down the long street that separates us. She has offered me food and rest and company until it's time to get the kids from school. For the few, long minutes it takes me to make the journey, I don't notice pain. The way is smooth and clear – not a single wheelie bin on the long, straight road. Oh, I laugh at that, after this life full of bins! And not a single person or a single car riding the kerb. I lift my chin and fly.

Each moment falls vivid and uncontested, like a touch on my lips. Dull house brick, tenacious weed, the flash of things enduring in the small, paved yards: cosmos, geranium, winter berry; green ivy flowers like fireworks. Spiky sputniks of horse chestnuts give way underneath me to sycamore keys then cherry leaf, blushing scarlet: a shifting pavement carpet, the air alive with the gentle spin of more. They land in me, resonant and whole and I don't think or shape them, I simply sail through, quiet and relaxed and altogether, utterly here again. It is happening more often now, this.

It is days like this that I remember again that there is nearly always something to enjoy. You can let it sneak up on you unaware, while your head is still telling you that something or other is wrong, even if it's right. The way the shoes of the woman at the pedestrian crossing turn up just a little at the toes, like wooden clogs. The plastic, jewelled hairclip, dirty on the gravel of Jude's driveway that I suspect rode the brow of a girl I love. The way my friend lifts her hand to her ear as she opens the door.

Look, here. The day is softening like a bruise. You are settling into your usual chair, and for the next few minutes there is nothing to do. See, everything, just for now, is quite OK.

I believe nirvana might be right here. I don't think it is just a comforting idea: I think it is a real moment, here and now, when you can drop down past the cacophony of thought and rest in what is around you. And knowing it is possible, unexpected and undramatic like this, waiting and open behind any moment at all, is the most enduring comfort I have ever known.

I got it all wrong, before. I used to think of happiness as a state to seize and sustain, but it's more like flashes that we hang in. It's a bright button in our vision to press, gently. To hold our finger against, just for a moment.

★

THEN

I felt it, this time, like an imperceptible narrowing. The rope around my waist was slowly pulled in, my world shrinking. It began to take longer and longer for me to get anywhere. I spent more and more time on the floor, measuring out the next fifty metres I would try to walk before I'd let myself sit again. The bird hide became an impossible distance, then the marshes altogether, then the graveyard. Each blinked out from my world. Soon, the idea that I had ever been able to walk anywhere 'for fun' seemed like a practical joke. I'd look down at my legs and wonder how I'd ever managed it.

I relented and began to use a stick again. 'Just for the time being,' I said. Within a few weeks, a second stick joined it, my legs dragging and shaking between them. I began to get stuck in places. On benches, on kerbsides. 'Are you OK?' became the soundtrack to my day. A ten-minute trip could take me an hour. Getting to school down the road and back twice each day became my entire focus. I'd spend the time in between catatonic with pain and fatigue, trying to recover before I had to do it all again. I dropped work contracts, worked from bed to earn the bare minimum we needed to survive. I was sure it was only temporary, until I realised it wasn't.

Jude drew me closer. She'd come over and we'd sit together and find ways to laugh at my shaky, useless determination, at the wild, baby-bird absurdity of my out-of-control body, and at my relentless persistence in saying I was fine, that it would all be *fine*. Some days laughing would turn into crying, and somehow we managed to laugh through that too. There was a lot of laughing.

'Right then,' we'd say afterwards. 'What next?' And then we'd think of something, and I'd face it. The day the mobility scooter arrived was a day like that. My maiden voyage out on it was to bring flowers to her house, in thanks, in defiance. I sped there, angry, jubilant, ridiculous, grieving, each feeling passing through me and past me like the tall houses of our streets. Her husband built a ramp to help me get up the step and we'd lower and raise it like a drawbridge, pretending to be pirates.

★

I have woken with a mischief in me. I blame the wind. It bites and nips at my face as I leave the house. It makes me smile. It makes me want to reach up and gather up a ball of it in my duffel-coated arms and wrestle it down to the cold mud.

If there is one grief left in me unresolved, it lies in my incapacity to be something lighter than I am. I want to be a being of laughter and play. A creased, happy wrinkle. A skimming stone, a weightless child. Instead, I am always so heavy.

It is hard to feel slow and light at the same time. There is something about slowness that implies mass, effort, restriction. There is something about suffering that does the same. Pain makes me sombre and careful. It shapes my mood, my face, my behaviour. It creeps into my words and my thoughts and my stories. It makes me focus on survival and necessity. I accept it, but I don't want it to be who I am. I don't want these heavy old bones to trick me into its leaden, ponderous suit, neatly squared pocketchief, ironed seams, and turn me into that forever more.

How do you run when you cannot run? How do you run through the day, clattering sticks against railings, kicking pebbles into gutters and autumn leaves into the air, jumping in puddles when you can't even walk to the bathroom? How can you be carefree when life is full of such pressing care? Be playful when you can hardly keep your eyes open? When there is no energy left for play?

I want to climb trees and sway in the highest, forbidden branches. I want to jump and whoop and leap. I want to lead you over fences with a wicked twinkle in my eye and get my knees dirty. I want to daub great canvases with paint, using only my hands. That's who I want to be.

I understand now why the very elderly sometimes pinch, insult and refuse. It isn't malice, it is the frustration of thinking you are boring and not fun any more. It is a desire to be light and to be free, fearing it is denied you.

I want to be lighter. I want to be an imp every day of my life. Perhaps the only way is to shovel joy and pleasure and play into my open mouth until I feel my toes lift off the floor. Perhaps I will eat joy like a child does. Perhaps I will start right now and roar at myself in the mirror or open my window at midnight and howl at the moon. When I eat my food, perhaps I will lick my lips and clap my hands and ask a hundred questions of the day.

I will learn to make slowness something full of mischief, I will.

A little boy sits across me at the community centre at a table with his family now, kicking his legs under the table. He has a pink milkshake with a red straw in front of him, and, look at that: so do I.

'Don't slurp,' his mother says, sternly.

I look at him. I look at my own straw like a winking eye, and I slurp it to the dregs with a suck loud enough to make the whole centre stare.

★

THEN

The big days landed quietly, unremarked upon. The firsts and lasts muddled until it was hard to tell which moments told a story of something ending and which marked a new beginning. I pressed send on an email to turn down my last high-pressure copywriting contract, closed my laptop and my eyes, and started to plan slower, quieter, riskier work. I began to advertise and write my strange, wonder-filled letters and then, a year ago, decided to write about my life. Was that an end or a beginning? What about the first day I pulled into the playground to surprised, uncomfortable stares, my son holding my hand, stretching himself taller with a loyalty so fierce that I felt the air crack. Or the day I first crept through the community centre doors, my eyes low, and found a seat amongst the elderly, comfortable regulars, emboldened by Jude's persistent encouragement that it would be good for me.

I don't remember the morning I learnt to sit up a little straighter on the scooter as I left the house, or the blossoming of an impulse to add lipstick and huge movie-star shades, but there was something of a first and a last in that too. The time I left confidently only to get suddenly, irrevocably stuck between a high kerb and a badly parked car and had to wait for help, a lump in my throat like coal. The day I called a carpenter to build the raised flowerbeds in my garden and took a seed catalogue to bed to assemble a new, simpler dream with scissors and glue. The moment I smiled at a young, handsome stranger to see him look me up and down with something like disappointed disgust and I knew myself recategorised. The moment it no longer mattered.

A new cardiologist had found what I had long suspected – that my heart didn't respond normally to movement and changes in position. Tilting me slowly from lying down to standing caused my heart rate to spike to 180 beats per minute and I couldn't stay conscious through its race. It joined a picture of wider autonomic deterioration – the regulatory part of my nervous system that was supposed to run my body's quiet processes smoothly and automatically. My feet and legs had begun to turn purple with blood when vertical, to whiten and blister in the slightest chill or flush and swell in heat; my hands sometimes too. Food passing through my body threw it haywire and the list of 'safe' foods began to grow narrower and narrower. Further deterioration in my gastrointestinal function followed, little by little, then my continence. New pains. New challenges.

I know that this is the part of the story where I'm supposed to punch through the page with a moment of redemption. I should have been moving you, all this time, ever closer, to finally tell you of the biggest day of all. An appointment, maybe, after all these new tests. A specialist should be sitting, apologetically pointing to an image on a screen, or a number on a list, and saying, 'This explains everything.' 'It's really very rare.' 'Of course, now we know what we're dealing with . . . remarkably easy to treat.'

The reality was, perhaps, the last lesson waiting patiently. My new doctors wrote 'dysautonomia' on my notes but shrugged like the old ones and suggested they see me in twelve months, reluctant to commit to much beyond occasional trialled symptom control.

My notes still ran with synonyms chosen to look better than a question mark: idiopathic, functional, prognosis unknown.

Chronic illness is a terrible narrator.

Invisible illness isn't an illness you *can't* see: it's an illness that people stop seeing. Their eyes slide off it back to the more interesting business of their own clamouring, confused minds, their needs and desires, empathy feeling too exhausting on top of everything else. I believe that is its own kind of unwellness. I believe there are many, many ways to be unwell that are much less visible than my own particular experience – some kinds we don't even acknowledge as unwellness at all.

'You'll have to learn to live with it as best you can,' they said, the 'it' stretching wide and vague and portentous.

And so, I did.

★

He has stuffed the footwell with cushions again and drives me around the world. I lie back, my legs supported, my twice-socked heels making little hollows in my soft car bed, and I watch, watch it all. We talk about everything we've missed in one another since last time, and laugh at each other, and let each conversation's association lead us to the next. I drift in and out of sleep when I am pulled that way and wake to find his hand resting happily on my thigh, the shadow of the forest flickering like water and the road clear before us.

We drive to Sweden because we can, over the Øresund Bridge. We eat chocolate cake and get soaked on an icy headland looking back towards Copenhagen, Fraser pushing my wheelchair into the wind as I shriek, happy, bundled up in my thick coat and scarf, tipping my head back to see his glasses rain-spotted above me. We turn the heating on the seats up to three and drive back across the country to Rømø island, across the causeway and right onto the beach, the hard sand flat beneath the tyres, and take photos of the wide, low light, grey and pink and still. One afternoon, we abandon all else and chase the sun as it sets, pointing the car down each narrow road that takes us closer. West, west, past potato fields, past goshawks flying low through the trees, until we rise over the crest of the hill and stop to watch it sink, molten, by a white, white church glowing red.

And in between all these things, we come home to the square, quiet house I am learning to belong in. We sleep. We slowly make meals together as I sit by the counter on a squat wooden chair. I am unwell when I am, but we do very little but drive, rest, and treasure the world, and so it doesn't matter. It is perfect. Throw a coin enough times, and eventually you will get heads and heads and heads again, all in line. We are old enough to smile at it, knowing it is nothing but chance and luck but something to be enjoyed all the same. Life is allowed to be happy sometimes, and often it is.

How strange it is. I have barely left the neighbourhood or my house for months, and now, when I do, it is back to here again. I was wheeled like cheerful baggage to the assistance desk at the airport – alone this time – and cried on the plane at the freedom of it all, until I was delivered safely into the hands of my love at the other end.

To come *back* is always a different feeling to the novelty of newness. I prefer it. I open the tub of moisturiser I left in the drawer and find the gentle impression of fingerprints. I realise, with a start, that they must be mine. Part of me exists here without me now. How could that be? How could I belong in such a place? And yet I know it and claim it: I claim each small thing. My son's bed, still made up, his night light on the bedside table. The jar of shells and pebbles on the windowsill that we collected from the beach the last time I was here. The splintered peanuts on the decking where I know the rooks feed in the morning. The bright rub and purr of the neighbour's cat. She remembers me.

'We will do all these things many, many times,' he says. I learn the layout of the local supermarket; I make up the fire with practised hands, and all I can say is 'Yes, yes please.'

After all that's come before, it has been disorientating to realise how much I have needed this relationship. I had been so sure of my solitude, wanting to prove to myself that I could go it alone, determined not try and fix my life by escaping into another. Perhaps what I needed, and didn't know it, was simply someone to be solitary and present with. 'What I want is . . . I want to be on my own, but with you!' I say to him one evening, muddled but trying as we sit with our separate books, and he laughs because he gets it.

How simple it turned out to be, really. Not complicated at all. Not to retreat from intimacy, but to adapt and explore what it could mean outside of any grand plan. To find a way to be with the right person doing right things; to move together with slow, honest understanding of one another and a shared appreciation for what is; to be seen and loved for the person we are on this day. This was all I needed and all I ever need. I lean into his strength and he leans into mine and we give each other the joy that we found harder to seize alone.

Oh, but this is a big love. We talk of it, still staggered. I am nearly thirty-seven and he is fifty. We have both read books and poems about love all our lives, but only now are we realising that the love they describe might not come to you young – it might wait until after marriage, after older loves and losses. And they weren't making it up: every word you've read about love is true. You might think you've reached the limit of it, sure the strongest moments of feeling are behind you, but they aren't. I suspect the same is true of all emotion.

We look at the decades we hope are left to us and wonder what on earth we have in store. Love grows, and my gaze grows, and my understanding grows too, and it all just gets bigger and bigger and there is no end to it, no end to life and everything it contains.

We drive up through dark forest to flat Denmark's highest point, and he pushes me through the mists and the twisted trees to the very summit, until the wheels start to sink and catch in the gravel. The chair abandoned, we climb the last few steps together, him half carrying me, his arm firm around my waist, and we stand and look down over the world that has been given to me whole this year, that has been given to us both to love together. The trees spread out below us in a vast, muted tapestry. Red and yellow and green, the fog weaving ribbons between them, the distant lakes hidden in cloud. 'I am so happy,' I say, quietly, and I mean it. He can see it in my face. It shines from me, up here on this hilltop, and for a moment, I feel sure I could do anything, weather anything.

How tempting it is to end my story *here* now, surrounded by all this, held safe. Is this not how stories like this are supposed to end? Finding redemption in the love of another, in the beauty and sanctuary of a landscape you feel made for, finally escaped from the hardship and restriction you've long pulled behind you? Isn't that how it should go?

Ah, but this is not a fairy tale, and this is not a story about leaving anything behind. I am still in the middle of my life and my story. I have a different, messier home, the vocation of good work to find, a boy to raise, and I love these things too. So no, not yet. Not yet.

I am learning that you must choose how to say goodbye. You must choose to fill it with the right intention. You must lead and let your heart follow. And so, we say goodbye with strength, with joy. With it, we mark what has grown between us since the last time; we commit to the next. We let it hurt, because it does. We do not try to declare it enough or not enough, but simply try to see its abundance, counting the additions we have brought to each other, that we've never had before. We reject greed with these goodbyes, or we try to. We try to embrace a quiet, happy gratitude. 'Nothing is broken!' he tells me grinning, 'so there's no need to fix anything yet.'

It only occurs to me now that we are practising – at least a little, at least for now – exactly what it means to be satisfied.

★

THEN

There began to come days when I saw that a life spent feeling this unwell was both more and less than I had thought. Through my journals, I realised what a gift all this solitude and stillness could be, that there are rich gifts hidden within it. I looked back at what had come before, the choices I'd made, the things I'd chased.

Maybe I didn't have to grasp or fight this time. I knew how easy it was to drown that way. Maybe, this time, I could choose not to lie down in my life, face first, until I stopped breathing, but instead put my feet down and bathe in that same complex pool and watch the shifting, humble hereness of everything. I could leave space for getting better, leave space for getting worse. Maybe I could simply enjoy my life.

I looked up and my family were waiting. Every few weeks, we'd set a date and all come together. My son at my side, who's never spent a day thinking that he didn't belong. My jovial dad, trying again, in love again, happy, with the beautiful woman we welcomed into our ensemble as if she always belonged there. 'Third time's the charm!' he'd say as his new wife laughed and punched him on the arm. My mum and step-mum bickered in their kitchen as they cooked the Sunday lunch, all bustle and kindness, and I'd sit with my brother – in his thirties too now, tall and confident and full of an easy, passionate joy that made me so proud of him, because I knew it had been as hard won as my own. I looked up and loved them all with a gratitude I've never shaken. I remembered that so much was still here.

I didn't know what was wrong with my body, but I did know how to care for it, and me, and how to care for other people. My life had finally taught me how. I wondered what else I might learn, could learn next. I'd write out pages and pages of bold, new thoughts and intentions, and then laugh at how much all this thinking got in the way of the main business.

The sparrows in the beech hedge teased, 'And how about us? Can we not be enough meaning for your life today?' and the twist of my son's hair at the nape of his neck said the same, and the fire in my mind did too, and finally I could say yes, yes, yes, you are enough today and every day and this is a good, good life.

★

I write this from my bed in an old terraced house. I've spent the best part of sixteen years here. Same walls, same view. I am glad of it. There is a difference between being stuck and being rooted, and my roots stretch down down deep.

I am unwell again today. How little that seems to matter now when there is so much else to focus on. How uninteresting it feels compared to everything else! Outside, the morning is cold. The bare lime tree in the gap of my window has emptied itself of its year; the sky, almost white, has too. My son phones from the school gates to let me know that he got there safely, that he saw a cat by the brook and found an elastic band on the path and Richard has taken all the skin off his knees again. He walks to school by himself now, a second-hand mobile phone in his pocket, his Head Boy badge bright on his chest. No need to stop and move the bins: his path and his time are his own. Some days, when he smothers the sofa with his expanding form, all limbs in over-washed pyjamas, I think 'I miss you,' and yet he's still right here. Some days it feels like falling in love all over again. How strange it all is, but then there are few finer ways to experience the relentlessness of change than motherhood, and with a catch in my breath and a flush of new pride, I am learning, I am learning.

There is a list on a piece of paper at my side: my plan for this next week. Stretches to do each morning; two books to read; a gentle schedule to write to; an intention to collect odd words from my day like flotsam, to write them out on small cards and make nonsense poems from their jumble. I feel a lift in my chest when I think of it. There is nothing better than something good to do.

When I came back from Denmark, the house was dark and smelt of cat. I opened the windows and put on another jumper and tried to let myself come home. I am beginning to think that beauty and happiness can break us as easily as suffering can. I am beginning to think it's all a matter of breaking apart and holding yourself still, whether you're happy or sad. When I was sick and unhappy, I could look at my life and see what I thought was missing and resent it. Now I have found good things, I could do just the same.

So many thoughts, so much consuming and waste and damage seems to come from a place of believing we're not quite there yet. That there is more, better, to feel, to be. I believe most of my life so far unravelled that way because I thought I needed to be something and somebody else, because I was desperate to fix the wordless problem that seemed to pulse at the heart of everything – or to find someone else who could – because I was afraid that if I didn't, I'd never get to feel right.

But what if I decided I was enough, and my life was too? What might I learn to love from that place? – everything? What would change then? This year has been an experiment in finding out. I think I'd like all the other years to be too.

I don't think the purpose of love is to make yourself happier. I think the purpose of love is to change you and to change the world around you. I don't think the purpose of mindfulness is to feel reassured or relaxed or to distract you conveniently from fear. I think its purpose is to *wake you up*, to make you brave and powerful, to make you a revolutionary who wants to live differently, act differently. I am not the same person for all this love and focused attention. I will never be the same again because now I know that what we turn away from will die; what we turn towards will grow. It's as simple as that. What a marvellous, dangerous opportunity it is. It could save us or kill us. It has saved and killed me in turn.

It helps to know that there is no winning here: that no one gets to win. Not at relationships, or mental health or physical health, or at environments or careers or at anything else. We must all just nurture and maintain what we've got, every day of our lives, and help each other to do the same. And sometimes it works and sometimes it doesn't and before long everything changes for everyone again, and that's OK. We don't have to hoard a thing.

It doesn't have to feel comfortable all the time, but it doesn't have to feel uncomfortable all the time either. There is room for everything: room to mourn, room to simply delight in what is, room to get better and do better, room for things to shift again and to start again.

Writing out my year has been brave. It spun, twisted and surprised as I wrote it out. I didn't know what the ending would be. Maybe someone I love would get sick and die. Maybe I would. Maybe I'd get inexplicably, suddenly better. Maybe Fraser would change his mind and leave me red-faced, heartbroken once more, poring back over these words as I decided what to edit out to save my pride. Maybe I'd lose everything or gain everything. The same is true of next year too. Now I know that I'm not supposed to know the truth of my life before I've lived it. The only way to learn is to try, blindly, to fail if failing is on the cards, to succeed if that's the draw, but then to look bravely at what I've left behind me, like breadcrumbs, before deciding which way to go next. That is why we must forgive our younger selves: we didn't know. That is why we must challenge ourselves each new day: we know more now.

Strength isn't about never faltering. It is about failing, about losing it, losing your mind and your hope and your way and yourself, but then one quiet day, soon after, making a new mind, a new hope, a new way, a new self – forming it from ash – and standing up and trying again. It's doing this over and over, knowing, every time, through happiness and victory and through defeat, that this isn't salvation, it isn't rescue, and it isn't the end.

Come on: let's not stay here. We don't have to wait to figure it all out. Let us bump our way down the stairs and cross the small rooms and open the door.

AUTUMN

The gutters are full of rain, leaves and the damp, blackened remains of fireworks: a late autumn soup. I wave and beam to the white-haired lady with her arm in a sling who still pulls back her net curtains every time she hears the rattle of my wheels on the path. Today she mouths 'cold' to me and hunches her shoulders in sympathy at my bundled shape and I nod and give an obliging, oversized shiver. I am back to warmest coat and scarf and mittens. My toes are numb in my boots. There was a hard frost yesterday that made the roofs white and outlined the veins of the beech leaves on the grass and turned the milk in the saucers that someone leaves out for the cats a pearly yellow. The automatic doors of the community centre whistle as I drive through them and half a dozen familiar, tired faces look up to see mine and they smile.

I pass the open door to the classrooms on the way to my usual seat. A girl kneels in a spotlight made by an angle-poise lamp and makes a silhouette on a white sheet suspended from the ceiling. Her soft, crossed hands make a fish, twisting, leaping in the light. A bird, a butterfly. She flaps its wings up and down and up and down, slowly, each movement a fascination, a choice.

Acknowledgments

To everyone in my life who I didn't get to mention or could only mention briefly: please know that none of this is a reflection of your importance or how much you mean to me. The hardest thing about writing a memoir was how many stories and people I had to leave out (or found I wasn't ready to write about). This book could have been twice as long and I still couldn't have done you all justice. I love you, the you who is reading this. Thank you for everything.

To the NHS for always being there. We may not have been able to figure me out, but for all my years of medical need, it has never cost me a penny. I am deeply grateful for that and don't take it for granted.

To the thousands and thousands of people on Twitter, many of whom have been following my story for a decade or more: your kindness and generosity towards me has been extraordinary. Thank you for helping me to keep going and for helping me believe I was, and continue to be, worth more than I have so often have felt. A special mention to Melissa Harrison and Simon Spanton. Both, in their own ways, gave me the courage to own the idea of 'writer' and made me believe I was good enough. I needed that more than you knew.

To my book midwives, Jenny Hewson, Alexa von Hirschberg, Allegra Le Fanu, Alexandra Pringle, Marigold Atkey, Sara Helen Binney, and everyone at Bloomsbury who believed in me and this book and worked on it so tenderly. You changed my whole life. It remains such a privilege to know you and work with you. Thank you for helping me to find the right words.

To the community centre crew for the endless poached eggs on gluten-free toast, and the cups of decaff (black, two sweeteners), with love from your quiet regular.

To my family: I am so proud you're mine. I have felt loved my whole life; what a gift you have given me. I love you more than I can say. To A—, too: I will always include you in this number. Thank you for helping me to raise the best boy in the world.

To Jude. The Legolas to my Gimli. Let's grow old and disgraceful together, yes?

To Fraser. Oh, my love. My joy, my laughter, my favourite surprise. It just gets better and better, doesn't it? Here's to every new day.

And finally: all things are relative. I end this thinking of the Millions Missing and many others who don't have the energy or opportunity to tell their own story. I am so thankful I was able to. It is all too easy for us to disappear. For those isolated, housebound, or bedbound by illness, please know that you are loved and that you matter. I am with you.

A Note on the Author

Josie George is a writer and visual artist. She lives with her son in the West Midlands. *A Still Life* was written mostly from bed and is her first book. She is currently working on a novel alongside exploring how drawing, painting and photography might help her to stay awake to life as it really is.

josiegeorge.co.uk
bimblings.co.uk
@porridgebrain

A Note on the Type

The text of this book is set in Bembo, which was first used in 1495 by the Venetian printer Aldus Manutius for Cardinal Bembo's *De Aetna*. The original types were cut for Manutius by Francesco Griffo. Bembo was one of the types used by Claude Garamond (1480–1561) as a model for his Romain de l'Université, and so it was a forerunner of what became the standard European type for the following two centuries. Its modern form follows the original types and was designed for Monotype in 1929.